MEDICINE
IN THE
QUR'AN AND SUNNAH

An Intellectual Reappraisal of the Legacy and Future
of Islamic Medicine and its Representation in the
Language of Science and Modernity

MEDICINE IN THE QUR'AN AND SUNNAH

An Intellectual Reappraisal of the Legacy and Future of Islamic Medicine and its Representation in the Language of Science and Modernity

Umar Faruk Adamu

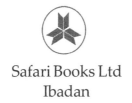

Safari Books Ltd
Ibadan

Published by
Safari Books Ltd
Ile Ori Detu
1 Shell Close
Onireke Ibadan.
Email: safarinigeria@gmail.com

© Umar Faruk Adamu

Publisher: Chief Joop Berkhout, *OON*
Deputy Publisher: George Berkhout

Published 2006
New edition, 2012

ISBN: 978-978-8431-14-5

DEDICATION

TO

THE ALMIGHTY ALLAH

THE MOST MERCIFUL, THE MUNFICENT, THE OMNIPRESENT

THE GIVER OF LIFE, HEALTH AND WISDOM

Contents

Chapter Three

Curative Medicine   **63**

Foreword 1

In the name of Allah, the Most Gracious, the Most Merciful, it is indeed my honour and privilege to write a foreword to this important book, *Medicine in the Qur'an and Sunnah*, written by one of our younger colleagues, Dr Umar Faruk Adamu. Over the years, a lot has been written about Muslims' contribution to knowledge in the field of the natural sciences and medicine. It is an undeniable fact that for over one thousand years, Islamic thoughts and ideas have held sway throughout the world and the legacy of that noble era was a prerequisite to modern scientific and technological progress. Dr Adamu has made a sincere attempt to tap into this rich Muslim history and bring into focus the unquantifiable contributions of Muslims to human development and advancement in medicine and other bodies of knowledge.

The opening chapter of the book was rightly devoted to the search for knowledge as the background and foundation of any meaningful human endeavour. It is shown that the Qur'an and Sunnah, the two fundamental sources of Islam, provide abundant evidence of the relevance of knowledge and the high regard that they attract from those who seek and disseminate them in the sight of Allah. The Qur'anic basis of preventive medicine is very well treated in Chapter Two. Aspects of a good diet, mental and social health and the strategy for the control and prevention of communicable diseases and epidemics are explained and brought into focus. The third chapter deals purely with *Tibbi Nabawi* (Prophetic medicine) in which the therapeutic or curative effects of certain natural substances such as honey, *habba-tus-sawda*, certain herbs and seedlings are given a great deal of attention.

In Chapter Four, the scientific basis of Islamic legislation with regards to the preservation of health is highlighted. In Chapter Five, the author deals with human creation and development in the light of modem knowledge and current research. This chapter specifically brings to view what the Qur'an has described 14 centuries ago which had only been "discovered" by modem scientists in the last century. In Chapter Six (spiritual health), issues such as possession, exorcism, miraculous healing, the use of amulets and the washing of Qur'anic writing off slates as a medicinal remedy, though controversial in some aspects, are presented intellectually.

The next two chapters deal with modern topics such as artificial insemination, family planning, abortion, immunisation, HIV/AIDS and so on. A lot has been written about these topics from the Islamic perspective, hence further reading and research is recommended to readers. The exigencies involved in some contemporary issues like the use of cadaver (dead body) for medical training, doctors examining patients of the opposite sex and the use of prohibited substances for medication are properly analysed. I find these topics very refreshing since they provide every Muslim with the challenge to possess an average knowledge of science apart from a basic knowledge in Islamic theology.

In the last chapter, the author traces the rich history of Islamic intellectual culture, without unnecessarily dwelling at greater length on self-glorification for past achievements. He also charges the leaders and scholars of the present Ummah to fashion out a course for the recovery and subsequent development of this legacy which has been lamentably lost.

This book, as an extension of other works, provides another avenue on the Islamisation of knowledge in the pure and applied sciences which need to be explored. I highly recommend it as a primer to those interested in the Islamic perspective of modern science and medical practice.

DR IBRAHIM MU'UTASIM, *MBBS, FMC (Paed) (Nig).*
Consultant Paediatrician and Chief Medical Director,
Usmanu Danfodiyo University Teaching Hospital,
Sokoto, Nigeria.

Foreword II

I have gone through this book, *Medicine in the Qur' an and Sunnah* written by Dr Umar Faruk Adamu and find it to be an important step in the right direction. He has used his advantage as a medical doctor to scientifically examine certain aspects of the holy Qur' an and the traditions of the Prophet (SAW) related to the field of medicine, and has presented them in an organised and very informative form.

Since Islam is the last divine religion to be revealed for the guidance of mankind, far from being a mere accomplice in this modem age, the so-called 21st century, it is capable of supplying antidotes to the failings and ailments of the present world. Analogously, this is also the aim of medicine as a branch of science, that is, meeting the needs that are most prevalent in the way of illness. This century has been characterised, especially, in the West by an increasing tendency to think that every domain of life should be made to conform to modem times. Fortunately for the Ummah, many of its bright minds along with Muslim scholars are struggling day and night to bring knowledge back to its proper Islamic axis. This endeavour in the Islamisation of knowledge – an attempt to reorient and recast knowledge to conform to the Islamic belief system and world view -could not have been possible but for the great dynamism of Islam which is reflected by its adaptability to all circumstances in all places and at all times.

It is in this direction and in view of the present circumstances that Dr Umar Faruk's work becomes an invaluable asset to every Muslim who values the legacy of Islam, and appreciates its contributions to the science of medicine for the benefit of humanity. The usefulness of the book is indeed very great. It cuts across region, age, gender or level of education. I congratulate the youthful and promising author for this good attempt to provide readers with the basic knowledge of the Islamic views on medicine. He has carefully carried out an intensive and extensive research on the subject. Apart from his background knowledge in Islam, his knowledge and insight in this field as a medical practitioner is, without any doubt, instrumental to the excellent presentation of the work. His ability to use simple and lucid language free from any complications or ambiguities calls for recommendation.

In a nutshell, the book is a step in the right direction. I hope it will pave the way for many more books on the subject, *Insha Allah.* I therefore have the pleasure to present this book to readers. I pray to Allah (SWT) to reward the author for the service he has rendered to Islam, Muslims and humanity in general.

Assalamu Alaikum Wa Rahmat-Allah Wa barakatuhu

DR MUSTAPHA IBRAHIM ADE,
Senior Lecturer; Department of Islamic Studies,
Usmanu Danfodiyo University, Sokoto, Nigeria.

Preface

A reference to the principles and practice of medicine in the heritage of Islam is in reality, a honest attempt to reappraise the contributions of the past to the present while clarifying doubts and misconceptions emanating either from a misunderstanding or genuine ignorance of the nature of Islam, its history or manner of operation. It is also an endeavour to reorient and recast knowledge to conform to the Islamic belief system and word view so that medical sciences (as well as other branches of knowledge) are channel to the pursuit of learning and scholarship that is of benefit to humanity. This was the noble tradition that early Muslim physicians strictly adhered to in the past and bequeathed to humanity.

It was against this background that the National Association of Muslim Medical and Paramedical Students of Nigeria (formerly Islamic Medical Association), a union of youths who are conscious and cognisant of their intellectual heritage, made a frantic call to branch organisations and professional bodies to attend its Annual National Conference and make paper presentations on varied issues addressing this challenge and aspiration.

This humble book is a product of such a lofty objective and a response to that noble appeal. The presentation of a seminar paper, "Medicine in the Qur'an and Sunnah," from which the title of this book is adopted, received warm response among all the participants representing various branches of the Islamic medical associations and other members of the community. Subsequently, several appeals were made for the expansion and publication of the research. This was my initial motivation for writing this book.

I was further inspired when I reflected upon the proliferation of various books, written in different languages, which erroneously presented some aspects of traditional medical practices as "Islamic Medicine." This is a dangerous trend, more so if we analyse further the implication it has on an uninformed populace. While this book is not aimed at degrading our heritage in traditional medicine, which admittedly and indisputably constitutes the foundation of the so-called orthodox medicine, emphasis need to be laid on the distinction between the two. Whereas traditional medicine represents the healing cultural practices peculiar to a society or community regardless of their religious affiliations, an Islamic oriented medical science derives its authority from the divine truth contained in the Muslim holy scriptures (specifically the Qur'an and Sunnah) and is therefore universal.

While making this clear distinction, one is also mindful of making reference to any body of medical knowledge as something intrinsically Arab or Islamic. It is observable from the onset that the book in both contents and title has tried not to use the phrase "Islamic Medicine" or anything with similar connotation. This is because, in truth, there is no such thing and there is no Islamic source that we are aware of, that subscribes to such concept. Similarly, there is nothing like Christian medicine or Western science.

Knowledge is the same the world over and, being universal, it is truly the world's intellectual property belonging to everyone. It has been so from the beginning of time because it represents fundamental truths. In other words, knowledge in its entirety, form and essence is a universal human heritage and no race, tribe, nation or colour can lay claim to its monopoly or ownership. This is a historical fact traceable in the memories of all preceding civilisations *vis-a-vis* their contribution to the evolvement and advancement of medical practice in particular and human knowledge in general.

The revival of the legacy of Islam in the history of medicine is therefore a genuine attempt to explore some of the scriptural references to the principles and practice of medicine in the light of contemporary knowledge and its representation to the global community in the language of today. Of course, Muslim scholars admit that the teaching of medicine or other disciplines is not the direct concern of God's book because the Qur'an was not revealed as a medical book or other secular disciplines. It is a reference material for a complete way of life in which God has cited for man all kinds of examples, pointing out all that concern man relating to his faith and maintenance of good health, calling upon him to consider the signs of creation and urging him to investigate further and contemplate. So whenever the Qur'an refers to these matters it does so in the context of guiding man to what benefits him in his spiritual, mundane and private concerns.

It is the primary duty of the Sunnah to demonstrate practically the appeal of the Qur'an. The Prophet's interest in the therapeutic, preventive and dietary aspects as well as in the permitted recreational activities and various social relations within an integrated framework that leaves nothing neglected and combines worship with health is based on the Qur' anic appeal. It is through his sound logical mind that he demonstrated the spiritual dimensions of health, role of psychotherapy, the relationship between body, soul and mind, ethics of practice, limitations and referrals as well as the removal of barriers across religions, races and tribes on matters of health and international concern.

One then begins to wonder the basis of the assertion that Islamic teachings underplay the nature of cure and emphasise the value of suffering. Subsisting that Muslims are encouraged to bear the pain and discomfort of diseases and seek the assistance of a physician only as the last resort when disease condition threatens to become incurable and pain unbearable. Some "experts" even went as far as saying that this attitude (to illness) is informed by the Muslim's desire for martyrdom or his inherent belief in fatalism.

Yet, a cursory unbiased glance at the heritage of Islam demonstrates the baseless of such generalisations or misconceptions. The numerous forms of herbal remedies, the many preventive prescriptions, the several curative procedures as well as the numerous prayers, supplications and invocations in Muslim scriptures overwhelmingly attest to the desire for sound health and the importance given to knowledge of the means to attain it.

The occasional reference to endurance and perseverance during sickness ought not to be misconstrued as a desire for death let alone martyrdom. It is a cardinal principle that permeates the entire teachings of Islam, medical science inclusive. Taken in isolation, outside the ambit of Islamic tradition, it may simply portray the suspicions of a community to a form of treatment considered foreign or alien to their traditional experience. This attitude has been a recurring decimal in all histories that showcase what is often referred to as "clash of civilisations". Thus, the importance of studying Islamic heritage cannot be over-emphasised as it will show every person with an unbiased mind the tremendous influence of Islam in the world scientific civilisation including medical science.

Those who reject the contribution of the past to the

present are simply and pretentiously being ignorant of the beginnings, evolvement and advancement of human medicine. Today's modern medicine is built on the best of the past. It is what it is today because it has drawn richly from the traditional practices of several peoples and societies at different periods of time developing stage by stage. The history of medicine is essentially a history of civilisation as there is no culture, race or religion that has not contributed significantly in its evolution.

To assume that modern medicine has nothing to learn from religion or other source of knowledge is not only absurd but is one of the greatest follies that cannot be reconciled with wisdom, objectivity and spirit of scientific enquiry. Let us not be in doubt that modern medicine in spite of its accomplishment and awe-inspiring progress has a lot to learn from religion. The scientific realm, which forms the basis and vehicle for modern medicine, is a limited realm and its world view is knowledge of a part, not of the whole of creation. That is why science generally, as a rapidly developing field, cannot lay claim to reaching its peak or attaining perfection. Similarly, modern medicine lays no claim to unravelling all the mysteries and phenomena surrounding health and disease or death and life.

Thus, a true reappraisal of the teachings of the Qur' an and Sunnah as they relate to healthcare would provide humanity with another reawakening and a solid foundation upon which a great renaissance can be built. Many would be amazed at the amount of scientific information contained in the Qur' an and Sunnah about the principles and practice of medicine, covering such wide areas ranging from curative, preventive to fundamentals of genetics, embryology, spiritual health and regulation of medical ethics.

This is the appeal of this book. If the goal of medicine is the objective utilisation of all beneficial remedies, as has been from time immemorial to the present, then this book would be recognised now or later, as a humble contribution to humanity's quest for better health and its struggle against diseases and afflictions, which recognises no barrier, race, region or religion.

Acknowledgements

For the preparation of the work, I am indebted to my reviewers for their intellectual stimulation and academic guidance, which positively influenced the outcome of this endeavour. In particular, I am thankful to the two sets of scholars, religious and medical, whose help I principally employed in order to provide a synopsis to this work. To them all, I express my profound appreciation.

I owe a special gratitude to Dr Ibrahim Mu'utasim and Dr Mustapha Ibrahim Ade for reading through the manuscript and also for writing the Forewords (I and II) respectively. I am no less thankful to Malam Tahir Malam, Professors Jafaru N. Kaura and A.G. Habib for their review and recommendations.

Among my reviewers, the late Prof. A. O. Badejo deserves special mention, who even though not of the Islamic faith, brought his vast professional knowledge and sharp objectivity to bear on the work. Regrettably, we lost him while the book was still under preparation on the publisher's desk. He shall forever be remembered.

I am also grateful to the International Institute of Islamic Thought (Nigeria Office) for publishing the work as one of their Islamisation of Knowledge Series.

I remain eternally indebted to all members of the late Adamu Dikko family for providing me with the foundational steps upon which this book was conceived, nourished, nurtured and delivered. To my teachers, religious and secular, who taught me what I did not know, I shall forever remain grateful. Furthermore, I thank Safari Books Limited, Ibadan for the very willing collaboration and ample encouragement.

Finally, my thanks are due to all those who have contributed in so many ways towards the success of this noble endeavour. I pray Allah (SWT) to reward all in the best manner.

> *Whosoever intercedes for a good cause will have the reward thereof, and whosoever intercedes for an evil cause will have a share in its burden. (Q 4:85).*

List of Reviewers and Editorial Advisers

Prof. Mahdi Adamu, Vice-Chancellor/Rector, Islamic University in Uganda, Mbale, Uganda.

Prof. A. A. Gwandu, Chairman, National Committee on Haij. Directorate of Pilgrims' Affairs, Abuja, Nigeria.

Prof. A. S. Mikailu, Vice-Chancellor, Usmanu Danfodiyo University, Sokoto (UDUS), Nigeria.

* Prof. A. O. Badejo, Head of Surgery Department, Usmanu Danfodiyo University Teaching Hospital (UDUTH), Sokoto, Nigeria.

Prof. H Ahmed, Provost, College of Health Sciences (CHS), UDUS.

Prof. J. M. Kaura, Director, Centre for Islamic Studies (C.I.S), UDUS.

Prof. A. M. Bunzah, Head, Dept. of Nigerian Languages, UDUS.

Prof. M. K. Abubakar, Department of Biochemistry, UDUS and Permanent Secretary, Ministry of Health, Kebbi State.

Dr Magid Kagimu, Senior Lecturer, Faculty of Medicine, Makerere University, Uganda and President, Islamic Medical Association of Uganda.

Dr I. A. Mungadi, Senior Lecturer and Consultant Surgeon, UDUS and UDUTH, Sokoto.

Dr Muhammad NMA Jiya, Consultant Paediatrician, UDUTH and President, Nigerian Medical Association, Sokoto.

Dr Ahmed Rufa'i, Consultant Gynaecologist and Director,

Hospitals Services Management Board, Sokoto State.

Dr Ramatu Hassan, Consultant Ophthalmologist and Chairperson, Medical Advisory Committee (CMAC), UDUTH, Sokoto.

Dr H. G. Sharubutu, Co-ordinator, Islamic Foundation for Science, Sokoto, Nigeria.

Dr Taofeek Ibrahim, Lecturer, Consultant Public Health Physician, UDUS and NSO, World Health Organisation (WHO), Nigeria Office.

Dr Bello D. Bada, Head, Dept. of Modern European Languages, UDUS.

Dr S. Khalid, Zonal Co-ordinator (north-west), International Institute of Islamic Thought (IIT), Nigeria Office.

Dr A. B. Kasarawa, Registrar, Department of Medicine, College of Health Sciences, UDUS.

Sheikh Isa T. Mafara, Chairman, Arabic and Islamic Education Board, Zamfara State, Nigeria.

Dr Jibril G Yeldu, Consultant Physician and Director, Medical Services, Ministry of Health, Kebbi State, Nigeria.

---

* Late

List of Definitions and Abbreviations

AS: *Alaihis salam* (peace of Allah be upon him).

Fatwa: A legal declaration made by a qualified Muslim scholar or jurist.

Hadith: The record of the Prophet's mode of life (that is, Sunnah) collected and narrated through highly reputable and distinct transmitters.

Ijma: Consensus of Muslim scholars on a specific matter not covered in the Qur'an and hadith.

Ijtihad: The exercise of judgement in accordance with the spirit and the general parameters of Islamic law (Shari'ah).

Qiyas: Analogical reasoning or deduction used as a source in the development of Islamic law.

Qur'an: The divine words revealed to the last Messenger of Allah (Muhammad) for the guidance of mankind. It is the first and most important source of Islamic teachings.

RA: *Radiy-Allahu anhu/a* (God be pleased with him/her).

SAW: *Sallallahu Alaihi Wa Sallam* (Peace and blessing of Allah be upon him).

Sunnah: The way or mode of life of Prophet Muhammad (SAW) including his actions, utterances and silent approvals. It is the second source of Islam: Sunnan implies plural for Sunnah.

SWT: *Subhanahu Wa Ta'ala* (Glory be to Him - Allah).

Taqlid: Blind acceptance of juridical precedent.

Ummah: Community of Muslims regardless of race, tribe, colour, nationality or lineage.

QUR'AN

We send down of the Qur' an, that which
is a healing and a mercy to those who believe (Q 17 :82).

O Mankind! there hath come to you
an admonition from your Lord
and a healing for the diseases
in your hearts (Q 10:57).

HADITH

Every disease has a cure. Knowing
the right medicine will cure the
disease by God's permission.

Seek for medical treatment, for Allah has
created no disease except that He created
its cure, apart from old age and death.

Introduction

Praise be to Allah, the Creator and Sustainer of the world, who said in His unique book: "We send down of the Qur'an that which is healing and a mercy to believers." May His peace and blessing be upon the Seal of the Prophets, Muhammad (SAW), to whom it was revealed and who commanded his followers to "seek for medical treatment, for Allah has created, no disease without a cure." May the peace and blessings encompass his family, companions and all seekers of truth.

> *Medicine is the science by which we learn the various states of the human body in health and when not in health, and the means by which health is likely to be lost and when lost, how it is likely to be regained or restored.*

Such was the definition of medicine in the opening words of the first chapter of the book *Canon of Medicine* (AL-QANON FIL AL-TIBB) of Abu Ali Al-Husayn Ibn Sina (980-1037 AD), the renowned illustrious Muslim physician known to the West as Avicenna. This definition (of medicine) appears to be similar to that given in modern dictionaries as "the art and science dealing with the maintenance and restoration of health, including the prevention and treatment of diseases." Yet, there can be no doubt that the intellectual framework,

1

the means and the methods of medicine have significantly changed with time.

Today tremendous undreamt of and astonishing scientific advances and discoveries have been made and are continuously being made. The history of medicine like that of law, is a reflection of the intellectual tone of any period. In ancient times, early medical practitioners were also religious leaders. They were healers of both the body and soul. Gradually with time, fields of medicine and religion began to separate and evolve along different lines[1] After this there was then an era of scientific enquiry, but this was at first dominated by religion. Subsequently, there was the dominance of science and the relegation of religion.

The monastery then was the repository of scientific thoughts and ideas. This was as a result of the crushing pressure exerted by the Christian ecclesiastical authorities on scholars and scientists who were propounding new ideas. For example, in the practice of medicine, the dissection of the human body was prohibited because of the "sanctity" of the body. The pursuit of knowledge in the basic sciences then

---

1. This was a result of effort of the Greek physicians in the 5th century pre-Christian era. The most notable among them was Hippocrates (460-377-BC), traditionally described as the father of modern medicine in recognition of his contribution to the scientific foundation of medicine. His name is also associated with the fundamental principles of medical ethics through the Hippocratic Oath, still sworn by new physicians to this day. He wrote many books on medicine, among them are, *The Book of Prognoses, The Book of Aphorisms* and *The Book of Opened Graves* (so named because it was said to be found when the tomb of one of the Greek Kings was opened).

became stagnant and Galenic[2] ideas, the dogma. The nature of disease was not investigated because disease was considered a visitation of evil and malevolent spirits, or a punishment of the Almighty for sins of omission and commission. Illness, therefore, had to be endured with equanimity and patience, and was curable only by prayer and intercession by saints.

The prevailing world view from the teachings of the church was based on an exclusive orientation to the spiritual realm that entailed the devaluation of the physical. Thus, everlasting life in the hereafter was considered a better goal than the temporary suffering of a temporal body. Celibacy and monasticism were sanctified and science and research denounced. The despotic authority of the church then went as far as initiating the Inquisition, a religious tribunal, which persecuted and tortured men of knowledge and new ideas; scholars and scientists were burnt alive or excommunicated. Ignorance and aggression were thus forced on societies in the name of religion.

This seeming contradiction between science and religion created a mutual hostility in both camps. Thus, when intellectuals, scholars, thinkers and men of science saw that the church was enslaving intelligence and preventing the free development of ideas, they retreated into a painful isolation from religion. Yet, the pressure of the church was not enough

2. Claudius Galen (129-199 AD) was the greatest physician of the Graeco-Roman era after Hippocrates. Primarily a physician, his 400 odd treatises included works on anatomy, physiology, surgery and pharmacology. His concepts, both accurate and erroneous, became canonised as the theoretical basis of medicine and surgery for many centuries. Sole reliance on the authority of Galen-"the sanction of Galen" has stultified progress in medicine for ages.

to douse the widespread reaction and emergence of free thinking and anti-religious propaganda which arose in Europe. These accumulating pressures finally led to a radical reaction when scientists revolted against religion and sought to recover their lost freedom. All the pains and anger they had felt found expression in a great wave of hostility against religion. This illogical desire for vengeance on religion led some scientists to the denial of heavenly truths and the existence of God. The ensuing spiritual crisis culminated in the separation of science from religion, the assumption that science is superior to religion, and that man is not in need of God or His guidance for his survival in this world.

This is the stage at which modem science and medicine seem to be at present because of the belief that all the problems of humanity can be solved through science and reasoning alone. But it is now becoming increasingly apparent that such a view is incorrect and that man cannot be viewed as a mere physical entity without a spiritual component. Along with this reality, there is the erroneous belief and stain attached to Islam and Muslims, that the religion is unscientific and retrogressive. This misconception emanates from the black and alien history of the relationship between science and religion (precisely the church), and the observation that Muslim nations compared to the secular states of the West and their associates are today lagging behind in scientific and technological advancement.

This scenario has led the Western world to believe that religion and all it stands for is reactionary, retrogressive, backward and superstitious, and that it has exhausted its usefulness and must, therefore, surrender to science. This opinion came to be the major characteristic of the Western approach to knowledge and its relationship with religion.

There is no reason why Islam should bear the brunt of the consequences of the historical relationship of the struggle between science and the church, and be considered retrogressive, backward and primitive. This is a hasty and misguided conclusion. For to take revenge on the church is one thing, and to hastily and erroneously have a prejudice concerning religion, is another. It is obvious that vengeance, being a purely emotional matter, has nothing to do with scholarly or scientific precision. In other words, so far as the Qur' an and Sunnah - the great sources of knowledge and inspiration - have not been adequately tapped, any judgement about Islam can be considered to be irrational, unrealistic and illogical. The era of persecution of scientists never happened in the world of Islam because Islam unreservedly encouraged research, provided clear guidance and enjoined Muslims, male and female, to embark on the sacred duty of the acquisition and the dissemination of knowledge.

Whoever cares to know about Islam will discover the fact that Islam came at a time when the whole Arabia was sunk in the depth of ignorance, superstition, lawlessness and backwardness, but it transformed that society into the most civilised and progressive part of the world. Subsequently, the broad Islamic world attained an enviable peak position through its unparalleled encouragement for the acquisition of knowledge (including the sciences) and its utilisation. Thereafter, both the state and the individual Muslim took the torch of knowledge to all parts of the world by establishing schools, hospitals, universities and other centres of learning whenever they gained political ascendancy. It is no exaggeration to say that it was through Islam and Muslim scholars, philosophers and scientists that the renaissance - from which the modern world received the gift of knowledge and power - came about in Europe.

It is the aim of this book, therefore, while clarifying doubts and misconceptions, to provide a thorough reappraisal of the intellectual and rich cultural heritage of Islam with regards to the principles and practice of medicine and its representation to the world in the language of today.

The Qur'an and Sunnah

Islam, as a complete way of life and the total submission and surrender to the will of Allah (SWT), does not leave mankind in this world without guidance. Such guidance is the holy Qur'an which He revealed to Prophet Muhammad (SAW) through the Angel Gabriel for the benefit of humanity. Through it, mankind is guided by many exhortations and explanations on various aspects of human endeavour, including the natural and applied sciences.

> *For We had certainly sent unto them a Book, based on knowledge, which We explained in detail, - a guide and mercy to all who believe (Q7:S2).*

The Qur'an is the greatest gift of God to humanity and its wisdom is of a unique kind. The purpose of the book is to guide humanity to the straight path and quicken the soul of man, to awaken human conscience and enlighten the human mind on different spheres of life. The Prophet of Islam had no formal schooling and he made no secret of it. In fact, it is his greatest credit that he was an unlettered Prophet *(Nabiyyul Umiyyi)*, rising from among illiterate people to teach the whole of mankind the true message of God. This is the first fact about the Qur'an being the word of God. The second fact about this unique book is the unquestionable authority of its content and order; a quality no other book of any kind possessed or is likely to possess. The authority of the Qur'an leaves no doubt as to the purity, originality and totality of its text. Serious scholars, Muslims and non-Muslims alike have concluded beyond doubt that the Qur'an we use today is the very same book which Muhammad (SAW) received, taught, lived by and bequeathed to humanity almost fourteen centuries ago! This is the book!

> *No falsehood can approach it from before or behind it; it is sent down by One full of Wisdom, worthy of all Praise (Q 41:42).*

The Qur'an is full of unparalleled wisdom and knowledge with regard to its source, characteristics and dimensions. The knowledge of the Qur'an derives from the knowledge of the author who could not have been any other than God Himself, who is the Creator of man and all other creatures. The Qur'an by virtue of its divine origin is addressed to all humanity, inviting man to exercise his own intellect in order to understand himself, his environment and the living organisms around him, both known and unknown, as well as to utilise those which are of benefit to him and eschew those that are harmful.

> *... We are never unmindful of Our creation (Q 23: 17).*

> *There is not an animal (that lives) on earth, nor a being that flies on its wings, but (forms part of) communities like you. Nothing have we omitted from the Book (Q6:38).*

> *... a detailed exposition of all things (Q12:111).*

This is the truth about the Qur'an. It unifies knowledge and directs it to its ultimate source - Allah (SWT). The knowledge of religion, of the universe, of man and other created beings are all gifts from Allah. Both the spiritual messengers of God, scientists and scholars receive their knowledge from God through many means and methods as He willed it.

> *Say: "The (Qur'an) was sent down by Him Who knows the secrets (that are) in the heavens and the earth" (Q 25: 6).*

> *And the earth will shine with the light of its Lord (Q39:69).*

What is remarkable about the Qur'an is that it embraces all the facets of human life from the simplest hygienic method of defecation to the intricate or complex advances in genetic engineering and manipula-tion. The Qur'an deals with human affairs in such a way as to give them a divine flavour and a moral touch. It makes the presence of God felt in all spheres of life and recognises Him for what He is, the source of all knowledge and guidance.

> *Our Lord! Thy reach is over all things in mercy and knowledge (Q40:7).*

The Qur'an, addressing itself on the guidance of man in the field of healing and cure, states:

> *We send down of the Qur'an that which is a healing and mercy to believers (Q17:82).*

And:

> *O Mankind! There hath come to you an admonition from your Lord and a healing for the disease in your hearts (Q10:57).*

And again, the Prophet (SAW) was commanded to make this fact known:

> *Say, (0 Muhammad): "It is (the Qur' an) a guide*
> *and a healing to those who believe" (Q41:44).*

In many other places, the Qur' an points out that it is a guidance and source of cure for all diseases (Q9:14, Q16:89) and encourages man to seek for the cure of all diseases and afflictions. This is the message of the Qur' an. God almighty as part of His infinite mercy and in order to convey His divine message to humanity, appointed Muhammad as His last Messenger and the seal of all Prophets to fulfil this need.

> *We sent you (0 Muhammad!) not but as a mercy*
> *for all creatures (Q2l: 107).*

> *We have sent you as a Messenger to humanity*
> *and Allah is the Sole Witness of this (Q4:79).*

Thus, Islam is a universal faith intended for all humankind, and the Prophet (SAW) has obeyed Allah's command:

> *O Messenger! Proclaim the (message) which has*
> *been sent to you from your Lord (Q5:67).*

From the above verse, it then becomes clear that the right path for man is that, and that alone, which the Prophet declares to be so. Thus, in order to follow the straight path, one must emulate the exemplary life of the Prophet which is based on Qur' anic injunctions. This is an absolute necessity.

*He who obeys the Messenger, obeys Allah
(Q4:80).*

The noble Prophet Muhammad has explained and
practically demonstrated the *Risala* (message) of the holy
Qur'an. The Prophet (SAW) was endowed with great
knowledge. He had a great logical and scientific mind which
enabled him to empirically advise the Ummah on proper
prophylaxis and prevention. He even offered advice on the
benefits of certain medications, natural remedies and surgical
interventions. The Qur'an confirms:

And surely you are on a mighty nature (Q68:4).

And the Qur'an draws our attention to this fact:

*You (believers) have indeed in the Messenger of
Allah an excellent exemplar (Q33:21).*

In many other places the Qur'an also constantly and
repeatedly declares that the Prophet is the "best specimen"
for the believers:

*So, take whatever the Messenger gives you and
refrain from whatever he prohibits you (Q59:7).*

Thus, the Sunnah of the Prophet represents the highest,
the most precise, best and truest form of implementing the
Qur'anic message. Hence, the authority of the Sunnah is an
essential part of Islam, and is second only to that of the Qur'an.
In fact, as the Prophet stated, both are inseparable as the
Sunnah explains and clarifies the Qur'an and, most
importantly, applies its teachings and methodology. Hence,
from the very beginning of Islam through the ages, the
Sunnah as a whole provides the stage by stage practical
demonstration of the Qur'anic injunctions in all affairs of
life, both the spiritual and the mundane, and has been

invoked and interpreted in the light of the Qur'an according to a known framework by learned Muslim scholars and intellectuals.

Therefore, Islam's pristine purity and authenticity is derived only from the Qur'an and Sunnah and if there is any contradiction or inconsistency between any of the traditions and the Qur'an, a Muslim adheres to the Qur'an alone and regards everything else as open to question because genuine tradition of the Prophet (SAW) can never disagree with the Qur'an or be opposed to it.

> *Say (O Muhammad!): "It is not for me, of my own accord, to change it (the revelation). I follow naught but what is revealed unto me; If I were to disobey my Lord, I should myself fear the chastisement of a Great Day (to come)" (Q10:15).*

And:

> *Nor does he (Muhammad) say (aught of his own) desire, it is no less than inspiration sent down to him (Q53:3-4).*

In an authentic narration, the Prophet (SAW) in his last sermon, said:

> *I leave two things with you after which you will never go astray; Allah's Book (the Qur'an) and my example (the Sunnah). They will never separate from each other until they meet me at the pond of paradise.[3]*

Therefore, the Qur'an and Sunnah constitute the first and second sources from which the teachings of Islam are drawn.

---

3. The *hadith* was collected by Hakim from Abu Hurairah (RA) and cited by Sheikh Nasirudeen Al-Banee in his *Sahih Jami'as-Sagheer.*

CHAPTER ONE

Seeking for Knowledge

1.1. The Concept of Knowledge

In Islam, the concept of knowledge is an extension of God's unity. God, according to the Qur' an, is absolutely real *(al-Haqq)* and not a projection of man's mind. The most important aspect of God in the Qur'an is His oneness. From this one God, then emerged one humanity which, though divided into races and tribes, male and female, is essentially one in its purpose on earth and in its ultimate destination. The unity of God, Who is truth, logically implies the unity of knowledge. This means, for example, that there is no bifurcation (division) between what is called secular and religious sciences, neither in their source nor in utility. God is the originator of the heaven and the earth and everything herein and in between. He is the Creator and the Teacher.

Who taught man what he knew not (Q96:5).

A critical observation and study of the Qur' an reveals that, it uses repetition in order to deeply imbibe certain key concepts or subject matters in the consciousness of its users. Hence, the root word *ilm* (knowledge) occurs seven hundred and fifty times (750) in the Qur'an. Thus, ranking it third in numerical tabulation and importance to the words *Allah* (God) and *Rabb* (Lord, Sustainer) which occur two thousand eight hundred (2,800) and nine hundred and fifty (950) times respectively.[4]

Apart from the frequency in the usage of the word *ilm*, the use of synonyms with many shades of meaning like *fkr* (to reflect), *fqh* (to understand), *dbr* (to consider), *aql* (to think), *fhm* (to understand) and *tbsr* (to observe) also emphasises the importance of this concept, that is, knowledge. Muslim scholars also tend to infer that the Qur'anic usage of certain objects or phenomena in oaths at the beginning of some chapters *(surah)* signifies its importance by drawing the attention of addressees to it and subsequently to the stated truth or evidence of the truth. These situations occur in several places in the Qur'an with regard to knowledge and its aggregates:

> *By the mount (of Revelation), by a Book inscribed in a parchment unfolded ... (Q52: 1-3).*

And:

> *Nun. By the pen and by the (Record) which (men) write ... (Q68:1).*

And:

---

4.   This numerical quantity does not include the other adjective attributes of God called *Asma'Al Husna* (the most beautiful name) and personal pronouns referring to Him.

And thy Lord is Most bountiful, He who
taught (the use of) the pen (Q96:3-4).

In addition to oaths the Qur'an also uses many words
that denote objects employed in writing and learning, such
as *kitab* (book), *raqq* and *qirtas* (parchment and paper), *qalm*
(pen), *yamuddu* (ink) and so on.

In spite of all these illustrations and demonstrations, the
Qur'an categorically and distinctly calls its followers to seek
for knowledge and dismisses any thought of equality
between the knowledgeable and the ignorant (Q39:9).
Consequently, the Prophets of God, who were the best of all
men, were all endowed with knowledge and wisdom. God
taught Adam (AS) the nature of the universe and the
resurrection (Q6:75). Prophets Lot (Q21:74), Joseph (Q72:22),
Moses (Q28:14), David and Solomon (Q27: 15) were all
endowed with knowledge and wisdom. Beyond revealed
knowledge - *wahyi*, certain Prophets were significantly
blessed with profane knowledge for the benefit of this world;
Joseph (Yusuf) was taught administration, economics and
astrology (Q12:6-110), David (Dawud), the art of making
coats of mail and other weaponry from metals - metallurgy
(Q20:80,57:25), Solomon (Sulaiman), the knowledge of
administration, judiciary and language of animals (Q27: 10-
20), Jesus (Isah), the gift of healing and cure (Q3:49) and
Muhammad (SAW), the knowledge of all professions
(Q34:28, 33:21, 65:11).

Similarly, the Sunnah of the Prophet is replete with
aphorisms and actions that corroborate the Qur'anic concept
of knowledge, making it the impetus and motivating force
for the future intellectual and civilisational development of
Islam.

1.2   The Importance of Knowledge

Islam recognises knowledge, spiritual or physical, as the foundation of progress. Hence, in Islam, seeking for knowledge is not only recommended, but is also a commandment or obligation. When the Prophet (SAW), about 1400 years ago, told a gathering of his followers around him that they must seek for knowledge "from the cradle to the grave" and "even in China," most surely he was not referring only to religious knowledge, but to the knowledge of the universe and the natural sciences as well. Thus, the efforts of the Prophet (SAW) were all directed towards leading mankind from the darkness of ignorance to the light of knowledge. To explain this, we go to the first verses which Allah revealed in the Qur'an, in which it is implied the constitutional provision for the acquisition and dissemination of knowledge:

> *Read! (Or proclaim!) in the name of your Lord and Cherisher, who created; Created man out of a leech-like clot; Read! and your Lord is Most Bountiful. He who taught (the use of) the pen. Taught man that which he knew not (Q96: 1-5).*

Scholars of Islam say these first verses by introducing the command, "read" twice, mentioning the idea of learning in different forms three times and speaking of the pen, which

---

5.   Qur'an chapter 95:4

is an instrument of learning, provide enough proof as to the relevance of knowledge. The Arabic word *khalaq* (which means to create) used twice in reference to the creation of man, also signifies the Qur' anic emphasis drawing our attention to the wisdom of creation. This wisdom is further highlighted in another verse where Alfah states: "We have indeed created man in the best constitution." [5] The Qur'anic description of Allah as the ultimate teacher, "Who taught man what he knew not,"[6] signifies further the unity of knowledge and its common source regardless of whatever names or synonyms we ascribe to it:

> *Is anything left besides error, beyond the truth?*
> *(Q10:32).*

Thus, in as much as Prophets are the spiritual messengers of Allah to mankind, so also at a different level do all scientists derive their knowledge from God through methods and means other than revelation, which only He knows best. Hence, the Qur' an harmonises knowledge in a dynamic and practical way. When the late Sheikh Muhammad Abduh, the great Egyptian Muslim scholar and thinker, made his commentary on these (first five) verses he said: "You cannot have more decisive proof put in a more eloquent way of the virtues of reading, writing and knowledge than in the way that God began His book and revelation with these illustrious verses." [7]

Commentators of the revised translation of the holy Qur' an by the late Sheikh Abdullahi Yusuf Ali observed in relation

---

6. Qur'an chapter 96:5
7. *See the creed of Islam* by Mahmud A., published by world of Islam Festival Trust, London, 1978, Chapter 2, pp. 12.

to this verse that:

> *The Arabic words for 'teach' and 'knowledge' are from the same root. It is impossible to produce in a Translation the complete orchestral harmony of the words 'read', 'teach', 'pen', 'knowledge' (including science, self knowledge, spiritual understanding) and 'proclaim'. This proclaiming or reading implies not only the duty of blazoning forth Allah's message as going along with the Prophetic office, but also the duty of the promulgation and the dissemination of the Truth by all who read and understand it. The comprehensive meaning of qaraa (though) refers only to a particular person or occasion, but it also gives a universal direction. And this kind of comprehensive meaning runs throughout the Qur' an – for those who will understand.*

Dr M.Z. Abdullahi, a microbiologist and former Vice-Chancellor of the Usmanu Danfodiyo University, Sokoto, commenting on these first five verses, said:

> *In these earliest revealed verses of the Qur'an is recorded basic and fundamental scientific knowledge about embryology and human creation; knowledge given to the Prophet (SAW) 1400 years ago about the growth and the staging of the human embryo, but which man's scientific research discovered only recently~ It is as if the Qur' an was saying to the Prophet (SAW) and by extension all men: 'You will come*

to know God through His creative attribute which is expressed in your creation in the womb and in all nature around you'. In other words, we know God, through the study of nature, and the study of nature (or God's creation) is what science is all about. The study of science therefore is essential to man's understanding and appreciation of Divine attributes. Thus, the first imperative of revelation not only underlines the necessity of know ledge for spiritual growth, but it also highlights the relationship between Islam and science.[8]

Thus, we can appreciate the fact that Allah, in His wisdom, has made reading the pivot of this Ummah. Islam asserts that those who have no knowledge are not equal in status (rank:) to those who have it (Q49:13); that those who do not perceive and understand are worse than animals (Q7: 179); that the meaning of revelation becomes manifest to those "who have knowledge" (Q6:97) arid "who have understanding" (Q6:98); that "whoever has been given wisdom has indeed been given abundant good" (Q2:269); that they deserve the right to govern who, among other things, have knowledge and trust in Allah (Q2:249); and that of all things it is by virtue of knowledge that man has been made superior to angels and God's vicegerent on earth" (Q2:30). This is the message of the Qur'an.

8.   *See Islam and the Development of Science and Technology.* Seminar proceedings (Series No.1). Published by Islam Research Centre, Sokoto, 1998: pp. 348-349.
9.   From Anas in Mishkat, 2

As for the traditions of the Prophet (SAW), there are countless examples of his sayings which show the importance of knowledge in Islam. In fact, the Prophet (SAW) was repeatedly reported as saying:

> *Seeking for knowledge is compulsory upon every Muslim.* [9]

The Prophet (SAW) also said:

> *When God intends good for a person, He makes him well-versed in the religion and such knowledge comes from learning.* [10]

In another place he said:

> *Seek for knowledge from the cradle to the grave.*

He also said:

> *The only things that one should envy from other people (if at all) are two: wealth expended for Allah's service and knowledge that is acted upon and communicated to others.* [11]

It is reported from Anas (RA) in a Baihaqi transmission that the Prophet (SAW) said:

> *Do you know who is the Most beneficent? Allah is the Most Beneficent, then of the children of Man, I am the most beneficent, and after me the most beneficent among men is the man who*

---

10. Sahih Bukhari transmission.
11. From Ibn Mas'ud in the *Sahah* collections.

acquires knowledge and spreads it.

Abu Hurairah also reported in Darimiy collection that the Prophet said:

> *Knowledge from which no benefit is gained is like a treasure from which nothing is expended in the way of Allah.*

Aisha (RA) also reported the Prophet (SAW) saying:

> *Truly, Allah has revealed to me, (saying): 'Superiority in knowledge is better than superiority in worship'*[12]

Abu Dharr, a companion of the Prophet (SAW), commenting on the sayings of the Prophet, said: "If you were to place a sword on my neck and I thought I were able to carry out one of the blessed Prophet's teachings before you execute me, I would carry out the one to seek for knowledge." Furthermore, fun Abbas said that the explanation of the words *Ittaqillaha* (Be God-oriented) was: "Be fore bearing and knowledgeable." Ali bn Abi Talib, recognising the importance of knowledge, declared it as "the greatest treasure." While showing the importance of knowledge in Islam, fun Qayyim in his book *Mifftahu Daris Sa' adah Wa Manshuri Wilayatil Ilmi Waf Iradah,* expounded and enunciated more than one hundred and twenty (120) aspects and virtues of knowledge.

---

12. Sahih Bukhari transmission.
13. Professor Hamidullah makes the interesting observation that almost all the Qur'anic verses in connection with knowledge belong to the Mecca period while the Medinan verses lay emphasis on its utilisation, action and performance.

All these show that Islam is a practical religion that does not encourage indulgence in idle spectilation and futile theorisation, conjectures, superstitions and fictions, and that Islam is knowledge in itself and all sound knowledge is Islam, for the two are inseparable.

Thus, the Qur'an directs man openly, and by inference, to seek for knowledge in reading, writing, research and its extension in all things that bring physical and spiritual benefits to man for the success of his life on earth.[13]

1.3   The Diversification of Knowledge

From the very beginning, Islam teaches that, in order to provide a balance between spiritual and physical lives, man should seek for the knowledge of both, which constitutes *Ibadat* worship.

> *Our Lord! Give us the good in this world and the good in the hereafter (Q2:201).*

The Qur'an recognising the diverse needs of man, encourages him to seek for all the good things of life.

> *Verily the ends you (mankind) strive for are diverse (Q92:4). But do not be negligent about your share of this world (Ql13:77).*

The glorious Qur'an has specifically commanded Muslims to engage themselves in diverse fields of human endeavour. It also promotes specialisation. Allah states:

> *It is not for the believers to go forth altogether for expedition, a contingent should remain behind to devote themselves to studies in*

religion and admonish the people ... (Q9: 122).

This verse provides the basis for the diverse concept of *Ibadat.* Knowledge, therefore, which is a form of *Ibadat,* provided it is genuinely meant for Allah's sake, is offered a special priority in the house of Islam. This is because it entails survival and prosperity and it knows no limitation or barrier. Of all things, it is only knowledge that Allah, the most High, commanded His Messenger (and indeed all believers) to seek for its increment.

Say: "Oh Lord! Increase me in knowledge"
(Q20: 114).

This Qur'anic injunction states no specification or limitation, but embraces wholly all forms or branches of knowledge that are useful and of benefit to man.

Imam AI-Ghazzali in his *Ihya'u ulumiddin* (the Revivification of the Religious Sciences), after extensive and intensive analysis of the Qur'an and Sunnah, recognises the unity of knowledge (in terms of its source) and its diversity (in terms of its application). Hence, he categorised knowledge into two, the sacred *(Shar'iyah)* and the profane *(ghayr shari'iyah)* sciences and stated as follows:

> *By the sacred sciences I mean those which have been acquired from the Prophets and are not arrived at either through reason, like arithmetic, or by experimentation, like medicine, or by hearing, like language. These sacred sciences are divided into four kinds, namely* **usul** *(the primary sources comprising the sciences of the Qur' an and Sunnah,* **ijma** *and* **athar**

---

14. Meaning the traditions relating to the companions.

Sahabah[14)], *furu (branches)*, **muqaddimat**
(auxiliary) and **mutamminat** *(supplementary)*.
*On the other hand, the profane sciences are
divided into* **Mahmud** *(praiseworthy)*, **Mubah**
(permissible) and **Madhmum** *(blameworthy)*.
And the Imam explains further:

*The praiseworthy sciences are those on whose
knowledge the activities of this life depend, such
as medicine and arithmetic. They are subdivided
into sciences the acquisition of which is* **fard
kifaya**, *and into sciences the acquisition of
which is meritorious, though not obligatory. The
sciences whose knowledge is deemed* **fard kifaya**
*comprise every science which is indispensable
for the welfare of this world, such as medicine,
which is necessary for the life of the body,
arithmetic for daily transactions (business,
'hlkkat, inheritance, etc) as well as other
professions besides. These are the sciences which
because of their absence a community would be
reduced to narrow straits. For if a town lacks a
doctor, extinction would overtake its people and
they would be driven to expose themselves to
destruction. Has not He (Allah) who has sent
down the malady also sent down the remedy,
given guidance for its use, and prepared the
means for administering it? It is not therefore
permissible to expose oneself to destruction by
neglecting the remedy.*

The Imam then cited the following verses to buttress his point:

And be not of those who are neglectful (Q7 :205).

And make not your own hands contribute to your destruction (Q2:195).

Hence, according to Al-Ghazzali, to specialise further or go deep into the details of arithmetic and the nature of medicine as well as such details which while not indispensable are helpful in reinforcing the efficacy of whatever is necessary, is however considered meritorious and permissible *(Mubah)*. As for the blameworthy *(Madhmum)* sciences, they are magic, talismanic science, juggling, trickery and the like.

Therefore, Islam does not only encourage the search for knowledge, but it lays emphasis on division of labour, diversification and specialisation in seeking for all the branches of knowledge for the benefit of man.

1.4 The Promotion of Medical Education and Health Services

In Islam, health and diseases are part of Allah's creation and for several purposes He subjects man to pass through these alternating periods of happiness and suffering. However, this does not mean that man should not strive to dispel diseases or seek relief from his afflictions. The noble Prophet was reported by Abu Hurairah and Jabir (RA) as saying:

> *Seek medical treatment, for Allah Has created no disease except that He created its cure apart from old age and death.* [15]

It is also narrated from Abubakar (RA) that the Prophet (SAW) says:

---

15. From Sahih Bukhari and Muslim.

*Every disease has a cure. Knowing the right
medicine will cure the disease by God's
permission.*[16]

This prophetic statement attributing cure to every disease
is a general rule that encourages people to undertake research
and understand the "right medicine" needed to cure their
illnesses. In exactitude, this is the goal of modem medicine -
the acquisition of the knowledge of diseases and the cure. In
the second part of the *hadith,* the Prophet (SAW) made the
recovery (from illness) dependent on the correspondence
between the disease and the medicament. Ibn Quyyim in
his *Tibbi Nabawi* (the Prophetic Medicine), commenting on
the above *hadith,* said:

> *When the medicament (mentioned for every
> disease by the Messenger of Allah) exceeds the
> degree of the disease, it causes another disease
> (instead of procuring a remedy), and whenever
> (the medicament) is in shortage, it fails to
> combat the disease and the cure will be
> ineffective. And if the curer does not discover
> the remedy or if a deterrent agent impedes its
> influence, then (in all these cases) no healing
> could take place, owing to the incompatibility
> between the disease and the remedy. But if both
> the disease and the medicament match together,
> healing would unavoidably occur.*

With regard to the above and in light of modem medicine,

---

16. From Sahih Muslim transmission.

we can deduce that the prophetic statement provides a pointer to the present day concept of pharmacokinetics and pharmacodynamics - the two important tools of pharmacology concerned with the effect of the drug on the body and the effect of the body on the drug - involve the dose-related effect, receptor concept and compatibility and body response. Indeed, this is in perfect harmony with our present day knowledge in pharmacology as a branch of medical science. Hence, from the above prophetic statement concerning medicament and healing, we understand the meaning contained in the divine words of the Qur'anic verse:

> *... everything will it destroy by the command of its Lord (Q46:25).*

In another *hadith* the Prophet also says:

> *There are two kinds of knowledge; knowledge of the body and knowledge of religion.*

By the above *hadith,* it means that the most important sciences are the religious ones which protect the soul *(Ruuh)* and the knowledge of health which protects the body *(abdan)*. The Prophet (SAW) encouraged us to strive to keep our bodies and souls vigorously healthy, for all kinds of good deeds can only be done with a healthy body. It is reported in several *hadith* collections that the Prophet, in recognition of the relevance of medicine which he referred to as "knowledge of the body," encouraged his followers to seek for that branch of knowledge. It is reported in Sahih Muslim by Zaid bnAslam (RA) that:

> *A man was injured and blood congealed at the wounded spot. The man sent for two men from*

Bani Ammar. When the two men came the Apostle of Allah asked them: 'Which of you knows more medicine?' They said, 'Oh Apostle of Allah, is the science of medicine any good?' The Prophet then declared, 'Yes, He Who has sent the disease has also sent the cure'.

Jabir also reported in Sahih Muslim that:

The Prophet sent a physician to Ubay Thn Ka'b, who sustained an arrow injury on the medial vein of his arm, and the physician cut the vein and then cauterised it.

It is also narrated in the same transmission by Sa' ad (RA) that:

The Messenger of Allah visited me during a sickness I had, he placed his hands between my nipples and I felt its cooling blessings in the organs that lie within my chest wall. He then commented: 'You are suffering from the enlargement of the heart. Call for Harith bn Kaladah.[17] He practises medicine. Ask him to take seven dried dates (ajwa) crush them with their seeds to form a medicinal compound and let him massage your chest with their paste.

The above *hadith* apart from laying emphasis on the importance of medical practice, also provides a pointer on the importance of specialisation, consultation and referral. Medical referral of patients to colleagues is indeed a desirable

---

17. He was a popular physician in Arabia at the time. He was to the Arabs at time what Hippocrates was to the Greeks.

and ideal requirement of medical ethics. Yet even today, many orthodox medical practitioners find it difficult to comply with this humble and noble conduct demonstrated by the Messenger of Allah, of recognising their limitation in skills and facilities.[18]

It is also reported in several traditions that the Prophet (SAW), in order to promote medical education and services, permitted physicians to take the material reward offered to them for their services, but he laid more emphasis on the spiritual benefits. Abu Hurairah narrated in a Bukhari transmission that the Prophet (SAW) said:

> *Whosoever dispels from a true believer some grief pertaining to this world, Allah will dispel from him some grief pertaining to the Day of Resurrection. Whosoever makes things easy for someone who is in difficulties, Allah will make things easy for him both in this life and in the next ... Allah is ready to aid any servant so long as the servant is ready to aid his brother.*

In another narration from Sahib Bukhari, the Prophet (SAW) said:

> *There are two gifts of which many are deprived, (namely): good health and leisure.*

It has been related from Tirmidhi that the Prophet (SAW) said:

---

18. It has been confirmed from authentic traditions that the Prophet (SAW) did not claim absolute authority on (earthly) matters other than the spiritual.

Whoever awakes in the morning with a healthy body and a self that is sound, and whose provision is assured, he is like the one who possesses the whole world.

In another *hadith* transmitted by Tirmidhi, Abu Hurairah reported the Prophet (SAW) as saying:

The first question that is put to the worshippers on the Day of Rising about the pleasure of this world is, 'Did I not give you a healthy body?'

Again, in another *hadith* from AI-Bazar, the Prophet (SAW) advised his uncle saying:

O Abbas! Ask Allah for health in this world and in the next.

In a *hadith* transmitted in Sunan Nasa'i, the Prophet (SAW) was reported as saying:

Ask Allah for forgiveness and health. After certainty of faith, nothing better is given to a man than good health.

In a Tirmidhi transmission; the Prophet (SAW) also said:

No supplication is more pleasing to Allah than a request for good health.

It has been reported that one day the Prophet's companion Abu Darda (RA) asked the Prophet (SAW), "0 Messenger of Allah, if I am cured of my sickness and am thankful of it, is it better than if I were sick and bore it patiently?"

The Prophet replied, "Truly the Prophet loves good health, just as you do."

The Prophet (SAW) also commanded his companions to explore and utilise several methods and means of treating illnesses and providing a cure. It is narrated from Jabir and Umar in both Sahih Bukhari and Muslim that when some of the Prophet's companions enquired about the permissibility of using certain methods of healing, the Prophet declared:

> *Whoever among you is able to help his brother should do so.*

In accordance with the Sunnah, Muslim scholars emphasised that it is an obligation upon the Muslim Ummah to seek for all branches of knowledge that are necessary or essential for its progress and survival. According to Al-Ghazzali:

> *The necessity to acquire each and every aspect of secular knowledge becomes even more serious if such discipline of knowledge has certain indispensable importance and benefit to societal existence, for example medicine. And that any community which fails to train a section of it in anyone aspect of these disciplines, such community could be deemed to have offended Allah collectively.*

In his *Tibbi Nabawi*, Imam As-Suyuti relates that Imam Shafi'i said:

> *After the science which distinguishes between what is **Halal** (lawful) and what is **Haram** (unlawful), I know of no science which is more noble than medicine.*

The Imam, a great jurist and skilled physician, was at one time aggrieved to see how much of this science had been lost by Muslims, and often lamented: "We have lost a third of human knowledge and have allowed ourselves to be overtaken by the People of the Book."

Sheikh Abdullahi bn Fodio in his *Masalihal Insani* reaffirmed that, "It is an obligation for an Islamic state or community to have abundant medical practitioners who treat the sick and the handicapped." It is against this background that the erudite scholar of our time, Sheikh Yusuf Al-Qaradawi in his book *Ar-Rasul wal-Ilm* said in categorical terms:

> ...*It is obligatory upon the Muslim community to get some of its citizens to specialise in all the various fields of human endeavour, to be able to teach them perfectly and also to transform and present them in their (hitherto) original Islamic viewpoints or perspectives, and in their Islamic garbs.*

Thus, in the book of Allah, the Sunnah of His Messenger and the consensus of scholars, Muslims 'are commanded and encouraged to seek and acquire medical education among other branches of knowledge.

CHAPTER TWO

Preventive Medicine

2.0 Introduction

It is the primary task of medicine to protect people against disease and to keep them healthy. The Sunnah of the Prophet (SAW) demonstrates that preventive medicine takes precedence over therapeutic medicine. The Qur'an and Sunnah, therefore, provide guidance on the prevention of diseases through the following approaches:

2.1 Personal and Environmental Hygiene

The Qur'an states:

> O you who believe, when you prepare for prayer
> wash your faces, hands, heads, feet up to the
> ankles. If you are defiled purify yourselves. Allah
> does not wish to place you in a difficulty but to
> make you clean and to complete His favour to
> you ... (Q 5:6).

In another verse, Allah emphasises:

> And your clothes purify and keep away from
> all pollution. (Q74:4-5).

In many places, the Sunnah also maintains the same encouragement and emphasis on cleanliness in its relation to good health, to the extent that the Prophet says: "Cleanliness is part of faith (Iman)." [19]

There is a narration that the Prophet (SAW) had established close relations with the Byzantine emperor, and that they used to correspond with and send envoys to each other. On one occasion the emperor sent a doctor of medicine to the Prophet (SAW). When the doctor arrived, he said to the Prophet (SAW), "My majesty has sent me to you as a servant. I shall treat those that are ill free of charge." The Prophet accepted his services. As ordered, the doctor was given a house and everyday they brought delicious foods and drinks for him. Days and months passed on and no Muslim (patient) came to see him. Consequently, the doctor feeling dejected, requested for permission to leave with the words: "I came to serve you (but) up to now no sick person has come to me. I have been sitting idly by eating and drinking comfortably. Arid now I would like to go back home!"

The Prophet (SAW) responded:

> *It is up to you. If you would like to stay longer, it is the primary duty of the Muslims to serve and show honour to their guests. However if you would like to leave now, have a good journey. But you must know that, even if you were to stay here for years no Muslim would come to see you. It is because my companions hardly become sick! The Islamic religion has shown the way to good health. My companions pay great attention to cleanliness. They do not eat anything unless they are hungry and they stop eating before becoming fully satiated.* [20]

---

19. From Abu Malik Al-Harith bn Asim Al-Ash'ari in Sahih Muslim.

By this *hadith,* it does not mean that Muslims during the time of the Prophet (SAW), or any other time did not become sick, but rather the promotion of personal hygiene, healthy surroundings and proper feeding are directly proportional to the health status of an individual or community.

2.2 Oral Hygiene

It is reported by Abu Hurairah (RA) in Sahih Muslim that Allah's Messenger (SAW) said:

> *Were it not that I might over-burden the believers I would have ordered them to use the tooth-stick (**miswak**) at every time of prayer.*

He also said:

> *Brushing one's teeth with miswak[21] is a good hygienic practice that purifies the mouth and pleases the Lord.*

Aisha (RA) also reported in Sahih Muslim:

> *Whenever Allah's Messenger (SAW) entered his house, he used the tooth-stick first of all.*

---

20. *See Islam and Christianity,* Waqf Ikhlas publication. No. 12, pp. 52.

21. *Miswak* is a short wooden stick from a special tree-Salvadora Indiea, which contains extracts that are used in a variety of toothpaste nowadays (*see* AL-Akili's translation and emendation of Ibn Qayyim's *Tibbi Nabawi, Natural Healing with the Medicine of the prophet.* Pearl publishing House, USA, pp.328-329.

It is also reported that he also used to brush his teeth before retiring to bed and when he awoke. Ibn Abbas (RA) said that brushing one's teeth with a *miswak* has ten benefits: (i) It freshens the mouth, (ii) clears the brain, (iii) generates a sense of well-being, (iv) dissolves phlegm, (v) fights plaque, (vi) prepares the stomach for the next meal, (vii) adds to one's merit, (viii) embraces the prophetic tradition, (ix) delights the angels, and (x) pleases the Lord.

Brushing one's teeth, according to Imam Ibn Qayyim, must be done with tooth-sticks of a qualified and a beneficial tree. Thus, one must not pick a *miswak* at random or from an unknown tree, for some trees are poisonous, and one must seek the particular variety of trees suitable for this purpose (particularly during fasting). Brushing with a *miswak* is good whether one is fasting or not, although it is needed most when fasting because it maintains oral hygiene and purifies the mouth. Amir Ibn Rabi'a (RA) said: "I saw Allah's Messenger brushing his teeth with a *miswak* while fasting." Imam AI-Bukhari also narrated that Abdullahi Ibn Vmar (RA) brushed his teeth with a *miswak* morning and evening when he was fasting.

Therefore, Islam promotes oral hygiene not merely as a religious duty or responsibility, but also because of its medical benefits.

2.3 Circumcision

It has been transmitted by Tirmidhi that Allah's Apostle (SAW) said:

> *Four traditions constitute the fitra (natural practices of the believers) marriage, cleaning of the teeth with a stick, the use of perfume and circumcision.*

Circumcision is one of the oldest surgical practices in the world and the legacy which religio-traditional medicine handed over to modern medicine. Medically, circumcision refers to the surgical removal of the prepuce (foreskin) in order to expose the glans penis in the male or excision of a part of the clitoris, labia minora and labia majora, in the female.[22]

Concerning circumcision, it has been proven scientifically that removing the foreskin of the male organ allows a better hygienic preservation of the area and therefore prevents infection. It facilitates sexual intercourse and eventually prevents the development of penile cancer later in life. Circumcision is of medical benefit in treating phimosis and paraphimosis (inability to retract the foreskin), tight frenum, balanopthitis (recurrent infection of the foreskin and glans penis). In present day clinical practice, circumcision is surgically carried out in order to secure a skin graft for the treatment of epispadias and hypospadias (abnormal openings along the penile urethra that cause the leakage of urine and the disturbance of the normal process of ejaculation). It is also indicated prior to radiotherapy for cancer of the penis. In infants and boys, in addition to some

---

22. In the female the resultant effect of circumcision is "sexual desensitisation" since the clitoris, which is the most sensitive part of the female genitalia, is the one that is removed in addition to other neighboring structures. Though the incidence of female circumcision is found to be high in a few Muslim communities, it must be pointed out that it is not an Islamic practice by way of prescription rather the cultural practice of some individual Muslim communities.

It should also be understood that in Islam, even male circumcision is not an obligatory but a recommended act and is part of the *fitra,* unlike in the Jewish religion where it is considered as part of the sacred covenant God established with Abraham and his descendants (Genesis 17:23).

of the benefits listed above, it is used in the management of preputial calculi (stone impacted within the prepuce) and problems associated with a long prepuce (foreskin) and in trauma to the foreskin (for example, fastening of the zip along with the preputial skin).

Of recent, a research work conducted jointly by medical doctors from the University of Melbourne and Monash University, Australia, revealed that, male circumcision offers protection against HIV infection. Using information from over 40 previous studies, the researchers suggest that the virus target specific cells found in the inner surface of the prepuce (foreskin). These cells possess HIV receptors, thereby making this area particularly susceptible to infection. The researchers proposed that male circumcision provides significant protection against HIV by removing most of the receptors.

The most dramatic evidence of this protective effect comes from a new study of couples in Uganda, where each woman was HIV positive and her male partner was not. Over a period of 30 months, no new infection was observed among 50 circumcised men, whereas 40 out of 137 uncircumcised men became infected - even though all couples were advised about preventing infection and free condoms were made available to them. Thus, the researchers concluded that:

> *In the light of (available) evidence, male circumcision should be seriously considered as an additional means of preventing HIV in countries with a high level of infection.* [23]

2.4   Other Forms of Personal Hygiene

Abu-Hurairah (RA) narrated in Sahib Bukhari that he heard the Prophet (SAW) saying:

*Five practices are characteristic of the **Jitra** (the way of the believers): circumcision, shaving the pubic hair, trimming the moustache, clipping the nails and depleting the hair of the armpits.*

2.5 Drinking Clean and Pure Water

The Qur'an states:

If your stream be lost (in the underground earth), who then can supply you with clear-flowing water? (Q67:30).

And We send down from the sky blessed water (Q50:9).

Abu Muthanna Al-Juhanni reported in Sahih Bukhari that:

I was sitting with Marwan bn Hakam when there came Abu Sa'idAl-Khudri and Marwan asked him: 'Have you heard that Allah's Apostle (SAW) prohibited blowing into water?' Abu Sa'id replied 'Yes, a man said: "Apostle of Allah, I do not feel satisfied with drinking in one breath", and the Apostle of Allah directed him, "Put off the drink from your mouth, take a breath and drink again". The man said: 'If I see dust or dirt in the water what should I do?"

---

23. See "Male circumcision protects Against HIV inflection" by Roger V. short and Robert Szabo: *British Medical Journal* 2000, 320:1592-1597 (10 June).

The Prophet replied: 'Pour it away'.

Imam As-Suyuti related a *hadith* in his *Tibbi Nabawi* in which Allah's Messenger (SAW) said:

> *Cover your containers and the mouths of your water bottle, for truly there is a night in the year in which a pestilence comes down and does not settle on any uncovered container without falling into it.*

Abu Nu' aim (RA) has transmitted the *hadith* that:

> *Whenever the Prophet (SAW) had a drink he would pause three times to take a breath,[24] invoking the name of Allah when he began and praising him when he paused.*

Anas (RA) also reported in Sahih Muslim almost a similar *hadith*, in which he said:

> *The Prophet (SAW) used to take three breaths, one after each sip and used to say that because of this it was more satisfying, healthier and more thirst-quenching.*

Imam Bukhari also transmitted another *hadith* wherein the Prophet (SAW) forbade taking water with a single gulp or when standing, and drinking from a container which does

---

24. The meaning of the phrase "take a breath" from the *hadith* is, drinking with pause for breath by removing the mouth from the container.

not allow one to view the water so as to know what is going into one's mouth, for there might be a leech or something else that may be harmful. Ibn Majah also reported another *hadith* on the authority of Ibn Abbas (RA) that, "The Prophet (SAW) possessed a cup and (water-skin) flask and used to drink out of these."

From the medical point of view, the manner of drinking water demonstrated by the Prophet (SAW) not only points towards safeguarding one from contaminated water, but also from the intake of clean water in the wrong way. The "pauses" advised by the Prophet (SAW) instead of a "single gulp," is medically found to be of benefit, as it prevents contamination by blowing exhaled air (mainly carbondioxide) into the water. It also prevents aspiration (water taking a wrong way into the lungs instead of the stomach) which can cause irritation of the respiratory tract, persistent coughing, chocking, bronchitis, pneumonitis, etc. Again, the Prophet's advice to "pour water away" once it is observed to be contaminated cannot be unconnected with his medical orientation and expertise.

It is now known that most of the intestinal parasites - helminths (worms), protozoans (amoeba), bacteria (vibrio cholerae) - which are the major causes of diarrhoeal diseases, dysentery, anaemia, weight loss, malabsorption, malnutrition, intestinal obstruction and so on, gain entrance into the body system through unhygienic practices dealing with drinking water among others.

2.6 Manners of Eating

It has been narrated in several traditions that the Prophet (SAW) discouraged his followers from excessive eating, eating while leaning and not to hurry to finish one's meal. The Sunnah also teaches about taking a variety of foods or drinks in one meal (which is our modern version of a balanced diet) and the use of the toothstick before eating, rinsing the mouth after taking meals, washing of hands before eating, the use of the right hand, handkerchiefs and so on.

In the light of modern knowledge, we now appreciate the scientific basis of the Prophet's injunctions. It is medically known that eating in haste or while leaning predisposes one to aspiration pneumonitis, indigestion, malabsorption, malnutrition and irritation of the respiratory tract. Similarly, many infections and diarrhoeal diseases are associated with poor hygiene, ranging from toilet care, washing of hands before eating to the actual preparation of the food, etc. Concerning overeating, the Prophet was reported, in both Nasa'i and Tirmidhi, saying:

> *The children of Adam fill no container worse than the way in which they fill their own stomachs. So let the children of Adam just have a few mouthfuls to strengthen their loins. If possible, one third of the stomach is for food, one third for drink and one third for air.*

The classification of the stomach into three in the above *hadith* is remarkably in harmony with our present day understanding of the anatomical structure of the stomach which is truly divided into three; the fundus (containing mainly air), the body (containing ingested food and gastric juices) and antrum or pylorus (containing mainly liquid diet on its way to the small intestine for possible absorption). The Prophet (SAW) was also reported in both *Sahah*[25] collections saying:

> *The believer puts food in one stomach, while the unbeliever into seven.*

Imam As-Suyuti in his *Tibbi Nabawi* explained that the "seven stomachs" in the above *hadith* refers to the divisions of the alimentary tract into different compartments - stomach, duodenum, jejunum, ileum, caecum, colon and rectum. Each of this has its own distinct anatomical structure and physiological function. That "a believer puts food in one stomach" is a figurative expression implying a caution against excessive eating to which all believers are supposed to comply. Moreover, the Qur' an likens those who are engaged in excessive luxury, overeating and merrymaking to ruminant animals:

> *The unbelievers will enjoy and eat as cattle eat;*
> *and frre is their abode (Q47:12).*

Imam Ibn Qayyim also in his *Tibbi Nabawi* reported that the Prophet (SAW) said:

The stomach is the central basin of the body to which the veins are connected. When the stomach is healthy, it passes on its condition to the veins and in turn the veins will pass the same to the body, and when the stomach is putrescent, the veins will absorb such putrescence and issue (the body) the same.[26]

> *Umar Ibn Khattab (RA) in imitation of the*
> *Prophet's Sunnah was reported by Abu Nu'aim*
> *(RA) as saying, "Avoid having a pot-belly, for*

---

25. Plural of sahih (a collective term for both sahih Bukhari and Muslim).
26. This is a pointer to the intricate process of digestion and absorption that takes place between the lumen of the gastro intestinal tract and surrounding network of blood capillaries.

*it spoils the body, causes disease and makes the conduct of prayer tiring." Harith bn Kaladah, the physician of the Arabs, was once asked: "What is the best medicine?" He replied, "Necessity - that is hunger." When he was asked, "What is disease?" He replied, "The entry of food upon food."[27] He also said: "The stomach is the abode of diseases."[28] Ibn Sina, the illustrious physician, also said; "Never have a meal until the one before (it) has been digested." Ali Ibn al-Hassan Ibn Wafid, after studying several Prophetic traditions on the manners of eating and the dangers of overeating, said, "Truly Allah (has) put all medicine into half an **ayah**[29] when he said: "Eat and drink, but not excessively" (Q7:30).*

Thus from the divine words of Allah, the noble statements of the Prophet and the consensus of Muslim scholars, overeating is condemned because all excess is contrary to the laws of nature and the guiding spirit of Islam, which recommends moderation in eating, drinking, sleeping, sexual intercourse, love, hatred, happiness, anger and so on.

It is now known that obesity is associated with many medical problems such as the obesity hyperventilation syndrome (Pick Wickian Syndrome), regurgitation, aspiration, pneumonia, chest diseases and low productivity.

---

27. Compare with Hippocrates's statement: "The maintenance of good health depends on working in moderation and avoiding eating and drinking too much."
28. It is medically an undisputable fact that, of all body organs, the gastro intestinal tract houses the highest population of micro-organisms, both commensals and pathogens
29. A verse in the holy Qur'an.

Obese persons are also predisposed to diabetes mellitus, hypertension, cardiovascular and cerebrovascular diseases, liver dysfunction, breast and endometrial cancers, sleep apnoea and so on.

2.7 Diet

The Qur'an encourages the intake of proper and adequate diet for the maintenance and promotion of health.

> *Lawful unto you are (all) things good and pure (Q5:5). Eat of the lawful things that We have provided for you (Q2: 172).*
>
> *Spend of the good things which you have legally earned and of the fruits of the earth which We have provided for you (Q2:267).*
>
> *You shall have therein abundance of fruit from which you shall eat (Q43:73).*

The Qur' an does not just allow eating, it restricts the dietary intake on healthy grounds.

Forbidden to you (for food) are dead meat, blood, the flesh of swine, and that on which has been invoked the name of other than Allah; that which has been killed by strangling or by a violent blow, or by a headlong fall or by being gored to death or that which has been partly eaten by a wild animal (Q5:3).

His statement:

> *Eat and drink, but not excessively (Q7:30).*

With regards to the verse above, it is made known that excessive eating can lead to obesity, which carries a high risk of cancer, coronary vascular diseases (artherosclerosis), hypertension, stroke, liver cirrhosis and a variety of metabolic and endocrine disorders such as diabetes mellitus and a host of other diseases as mentioned earlier.

The drinks which Islam considers harmful are included in the Qur'anic verse, which forbids all intoxicants including alcohol, hard drugs and drug abuse (Q5:93-94). Alcohol consumption is now known to increase the incidence of several cancers and inflammatory conditions of the gastro-intestinal tract, liver cirrhosis, pancreatitis, cardiomyopathies and various disorders of the central and peripheral nervous systems.

With regards to cigarette smoking, several studies have established its association with the development of cancers in many organs of the body, particularly the lungs and the bladder. Cigarette smoke is known to contain an estimated 4,000 chemicals, which are cytotoxic, mutogenic, antigenic and carcinogenic. Smoking causes the irritation of the respiratory epithelium, poor pulmonary compliance, respiratory failure and is known to enhance thrombosis, anaemia, and delays the healing of gastro-duodenal ulcers. Smoking is now known to be associated with the high incidence of coronary heart disease, cardiomyopathies, artherosclerosis and congenital abnormalities.

The general principle of the Qur'an and Sunnah in diet regulation and restriction is therefore very clear.

All things which are pure in themselves and good for man are lawful for diet as long as they are taken in moderate quantities. And all the things which are impure and bad or harmful are unlawful under all ordinary circumstances. However, there is always room and flexibility for exceptions to meet cases of absolute necessity (Q2: 173,5:5).

2.8 Physical Health - Sport, Amusement and Recreation

It is gratifying to notice that most of the Islamic forms of worship, for example, prayer, pilgrimage, fasting, etc display some sportive characteristics, although they are basically and by nature meant for spiritual purposes. But who could deny the constant interaction between the physique and the morale of man? For the improvement of the physical condition of the individual in addition to controlling anxiety, depression and other emotional problems, sportive activities and amusements are encouraged so long as they do not anticipate or involve sin, or cause any harm or delay or hamper the fulfilment of other obligations.

> Say: *Who has forbidden the beautiful (gifts) of Allah which He has produced for His servants and the things clean and pure which He has provided for sustenance? (Q7:32).*

The Prophet (SAW) told one of his companions who keep away from the common life and amusement and remain fully devoted to prayers and fasting, " ... there is time for this and a time for that." He repeated the phrase three times (referring to the balance between *Ibadat* and recreational activities). [30]

Following the Prophet's example, his noble and pious companions also enjoyed humour, laughter, play and sport, which relaxed their bodies and minds. Ali bn Abi Talib (RA) said:

> *Minds get tired as bodies do, so treat them with humour and refresh your minds from time to*

time, for a tired mind becomes blind.

Another famous Prophet's companion, Abu Al-Darda (RA) said:

> *I entertain my heart with something trivial in order to make it stronger in the service of truth.*

In another *hadith* Abdullah bn Amr (RA) reported that:

> *The Messenger of Allah (SAW) said to me, O Abdullahi! Am I not told that you fast in the day time and stand up in devotion during the night?" I said, 'Yes, O Messenger of Allah', He (then) said: 'Do not do so, keep fast and break: it and stand up in devotion (in the night) and have sleep, for your body, your eyes, your wife, and your visitor (guest) has a right over you.* [31]

Accordingly, a Muslim can entertain himself in order to relax his mind or refresh himself with permissible sport or play with his friends. However, it is a regrettable mistake to associate with sports and amusements, things which are not really sportive or amusing. Some people consider gambling, nudity, sex and alcohol as sports and amusements, but this is not the view point of Islam.

> *Is the one who is on a clear path from his Lord, no better than one to whom the evil of his conduct seems pleasing, and as such follow their own lusts? (Q47: 14).* [32]

30. Cited in Qaradawi's *Halal wal Haram Fil-islam*.
31. Sahih Bukhari transmission.

On the issue of music, which is part of recreational activities, several Islamic scholars have addressed themselves to its restriction, but have never outrightly regarded it as prohibited except where it is associated with certain disapproved behaviour (like idleness, nudity, dissoluteness, slander, etc).

Other Components of Health

With reference to the definition of health by the World Health Organisa-tion (WHO)[33] in its constitution as "a state of complete physical, mental and social well-being and not merely the absence of diseases and infirmity," the Qur' an and Sunnah gives the following guidelines:

2.9 Social Health

The Qur'an states:

> O mankind, fear your lord Who created you all
> from a single soul and from it He created its
> mate and from them scattered multitudes of men
> and women. Fear Allah ... verily Allah has been
> a Watcher over you (Q4: 1).

---

32. This verse is comparable to the Biblical statement, "To the stupid one the carrying of loose conduct is like sport," (Proverbs 10:23).
33. WHO is an international, Intergovernmental organisation forming part of the United Nation system, with the aim of "the attainment by all peoples of the highest possible level of health." It is concerned in particular with major problems the solutions of which call for the co-operation of many countries, such as the campaign against trans-missible diseases, cancer and cardiovascular diseases. It also lays down international standards for biologic preparations and norms, maintains international health regulations, disseminates epidemio-logic information (for planning of health services) and encourages research and the exchange of scientific knowledge. It has an impor-tant role in the standardisation of terminology in the health field.

Sexual promiscuity, homosexuality, sexual intercourse during menstruation, etc are all forbidden in Islam (Q.23:5, 24:30, 70:29). All these vices are associated with the high incidence of venereal or sexually transmitted diseases (STDs), cancers, infertility, inflammatory diseases and the most dreaded Human Immunodeficiency Virus (HIV) infection or Acquired Immunodeficiency Syndrome (AIDS). Smoking, alcohol consumption, the attendance of movies or cinema that display nudity and sex scenes are all condemned by Allah (Q.17:26, 11:15,5:93). The Qur'an warns:

> *And spend your wealth in the course of Allah and make not your own hands contribute to (your) destruction (Q2:195).*

Islam stands for human welfare and recognises that you have a certain right upon you. Islam enjoins man the use of all clean, healthy and useful things and asks him not to deprive his body of clean foods and drinks. Islam does not believe in the suppression of sexual desire, it enjoins man to control and regulate it and seek its fulfllment in marriage. It forbids him to resort to self-persecution and total self-denial and permits him to enjoy the rightful comforts and pleasures of life and remain pious and steadfast. It exhorts him to work for a living and strongly disapproves idleness, joblessness and begging. Islam also bids him to recognise the rights of others, the aged, the child, the woman and other members of the society and to respect the law.

> *He (Allah) has not laid upon you in religion any hardship (Q22:78).*

Accordingly, the Prophet (SAW) said, "Eat, drink, wear clothes and give alms without extravagance and without conceit." Ibn Abbas also said, "Eat what you wish and wear what you wish, if you can avoid extravagance and conceit."[34]

It is reported by Jabir (RA) that the Prophet (SAW) said, "Whoever among you is troubled by his sexual urge, let him marry, for marriage causes the eyes to be lowered and safeguards the private parts." [35] He also advised one of his companions, "Go and take a virgin as your wife whom you will caress and who will caress you." It is reported in several traditions that the Prophet (SAW) advised his companions to wash themselves after sexual intimacy (intercourse) and to avoid coitus with their wives while lacking desire, or when they are sick or dirty. He also encouraged foreplay (caressing) before love-making. The Prophet (SAW) also condemned anal sex, but allowed any position provided the vagina is used.

> *Permitted to you is the approach to your wives.*
> *They are your garments and you their garments*
> *(Q2: 187).*

And:

> *Your wives are as a tilth unto you, so approach*
> *your tilth when or how you will (Q2:223).*

Concerning the choice of a marriage partner, the Prophet (SAW) mentioned in the *Sahah* collections, "A woman is taken as a bride for her fortune, her honourable lineage, her beauty or her devotion. Marry the pious woman or else your hand will become destitute." Again, Islam permits (not commands)

---

34. Collected by Sahih Bukhari and cited by Yusufu AL-Qaradawi in his *Al-Sahwa al Islamiyah bayna al Juhud wa al Tatarruf.*
35. Note that in certain circumstance Islam permits celibacy to one who can adequately control his sexual urge

a Muslim to marry more than one wife if the need arises, because it is compatible with the law of human nature:

> *Marry women of your choice, two, or three or four; but if you fear that you shall not be able to deal justly (with them), then marry only one (Q4:3).*

From the above Prophetic and Qur'anic statements, it is made clear that, the Islamic mission aims to refme, guide and control the human instincts and to purge them of all perversions and excesses, but not to annihilate or abolish them, for this does not represent the logic of a true religion. Some people think: that religion is against all enjoyment and is in no mood to compromise with the pleasures of this world, as if God is forcing man to choose between the happiness in this world and the happiness in the hereafter, thereby condemning him to enduring one of the two forms of misery. In contrast, Islam teaches that, it is entirely possible to combine happiness in this world with happiness in the hereafter.

> *Our Lord! Give us the good in this world and the good in the hereafter (Q2:201).*

Medically, it is known that a fruitful existence for man is dependent on the active presence in his life of the deployment of his instincts in proper equilibrium. The suppression of these instincts leads to complexes and the destruction of the personality, leading to social breakdown and psychological disorders. The sexual instinct, according to Sigmund Freud, is one of the greatest of human instincts. Again, since human beings differ in their physiological and biological variables, the Islamic flexible approach of permitting celibacy, monogamy and polygamy at different stages and varying circumstances, is deeply rooted upon the knowledge of medical science.

Pertaining to the *hadith*, which recommends foreplay before coitus, caressing is medically found to be beneficial for both partners, as it arouses desire, relaxes the mind, reduces tension, allays fear and apprehension and stimulates secretions, which moisten the vagina and allow easy passage of the penis. Caressing, therefore, is a medical treatment for frigidity, vaginismus, [36] dyspareunia (painful sexual intercourse) and the prevention of post-coital bleeding and bruises secondary to trauma and anxiety, which can mar a marriage and promote suspicion and hatred.

The Islamic stand also on hard drugs, drug abuse and intoxicants is distinct and clear - "whatever intoxicates is prohibited even in small amounts." This is one of the most formidable preventive measures against drug dependence, abuse and addiction, which ought to be adopted by the World Health Organisation.[37]

2.10 Mental Health

The most important' guidance on the mental health is the belief in Allah (SWT), His destiny and power over all creatures and things. The lack of recognition of Allah as the ultimate source of sustenance, relief, protection, support and guidance can easily lead to anxiety, depression and a host of other mental illnesses.

Concerning those who are doubtful or suspicious of the solid fact regarding the Lordship of Allah (SWA), the Qur'an

---

36. Spasms of the perivaginal muscles, there making sexual intercourse or penetration impossible and painful

states:

> *In their hearts is a disease and Allah has caused their sickness to intensify (Q2: 10).*

He also said:

> *Whosoever turns away from My message, verily for him is a life narrowed down (Q20: 124).*

On the other hand:

> *He who gives (in charity) and fears (Allah), We will indeed make smooth for him the path of ease (Q92:7).*

Thus, belief in Allah and reliance on Him reduce or eliminate the risk of mental illness, hypertension, stress, anxiety, psychological breakdown and a tormenting conscience. Abu Said Al-Khudri and Abu Hurairah narrated in both the Sahah collections that the Messenger of Allah (SAW) said:

> *No fatigue, nor disease, nor sorrow, nor sadness, nor hurt, nor distress befalls a Muslim even if it were the prick he receives from a thorn but that Allah expiates some of his sins for that.*

In Islam, patience is the key to relief from the stresses of life and is an indication of faith and the certainty of belief. Trials, tests and tribulations are part of life, and a Muslim is expected to understand this fact and try to adapt to it. We

---

37. Consider the outcry of the UN Secretary, Kofi Annan, "Drugs are tearing apart our societies, spawning crime, spreading diseases such as AIDS, and killing our youth and our future. Today there are an estimated 190 million drug users around the world" (See Awake! November 8, 1999).

have already been forewarned:

> *We shall certainly test you with a certain amount of fear and hunger and loss of wealth and life and fruits. But give glad tidings to the steadfast, who say, when afflicted with calamity: "To Allah we belong, and to Him is our return"* *(Q2: 155-156).*

The Prophet (SAW) was reported by Abu Hurairah in Sahib Bukhari as saying, "If Allah wants to do good to somebody, He afflicts him with trials."

Thus, Islam teaches that, though emotions such as anger, anxiety, sorrow, shame and joy are natural instincts, man must try to control them within healthy limits. The Prophet (SAW) was once asked for word of advice and he repeatedly replied, "Never be angry."[38] And this is the meaning of the statement of the Almighty, "Those who restrain their anger and pardon all men" (Q3: 134). Hence, regarding grief, anxiety and sorrow, the Prophet (SAW) used to seek refuge in Allah at the end of every prayer in order to escape them. The Prophet (SAW) also recommended prayer, exercise, *wudu* (ablution) and sleep when someone is in distress or trials. The Qur'an states:

> *No misfortune can happen on earth or in your soul but is recorded in a book before We bring it into existence, ... (so) despair not over matters that pass you by (Q57:22).*

As for joy or happiness, its characteristic is to strengthen inward energy and improve body's immune status. Allah states:

> Say: *In the outpouring generosity of Allah, and in His mercy, - in that, let them rejoice (Q10:58).*

However, even happiness, if it is excessive, can be self-destructive.

> *Exult not, for Allah loveth not those who exult (Q28:76).*

The Qur'an emphasises again:

> *Exult not over favours bestowed upon you. For Allah loveth not any vainglorious boaster (Q57:23).*

Therefore, in whatever circumstance and predicament a believer finds himself, Islam encourages him to turn to Allah and have total and complete faith in Him. The same (faith and devotion) is also expected from the patient's relatives or caretakers.

> *Never give up hope of Allah's soothing mercy; truly no one despairs of Allah's mercy, except those who have no faith (Q12:87).*

2.11 The Control of Communicable Diseases and Epidemics

The Prophet (SAW) was reported by both Sa' ad and Ibn Abbas (RA saying:

> *If you hear an epidemic has broken out in a land do not go into it, and if it occurs in a land while you were there, do not flee from it.*[39]

---

38. From Abu Hurairah (RA) in Bukhari transmission.

It was on account of the above *hadith*, that Umar bn Khattab (RA), as the Caliph of the Muslims, while on an official trip with an entourage to Syria, cancelled his journey after being informed that an epidemic had broken out there. When he was confronted by Abu Ubaidah bin Al-Jarrah, "Are you running away from the decree of Allah?" Vmar wisely replied, "O Abu Ubaidah! Yes, we are running away from the decree of Allah to the decree of Allah."[40]

In Islam, falling victim to a pestilence happens according to the decree of Allah and seeking protection from that by using medicine and adopting other preventing measures in order to save oneself from it, is also within the orbit of divine decree. This is exactly what Caliph Umar meant by his statement, "from the decree of Allah to the decree of Allah."

In a *hadith* reported by Abu Hurairah in Sahih Bukhari collection, the Prophet (SAW) said, "Do not put (in the same room) a sick person with a healthy person." In a Sahih Muslim transmission, he also said, "Let the carrier of an infectious disease not visit a healthy person."

From the above *hadith* of the Prophet (SAW) concerning the possibility of the transmission of certain diseases and the measures or precautions to take, we can appreciate the fact that the present approach of modem medicine is not different from it. In short, the concept of quarantine, the isolation unit, hospital construction, barrier nursing or management, the use of gloves and protective wear, the sterilisation of instruments and so on, are all geared towards preventing the spread of nasocomial infections and epidemic or pandemic outbreak.[41]

---

39. Sahih Bukhari and Muslim transmission.
40. This *hadith* was reported by Abdullahi Ibn Abbas and Abdullahi bn Amir and is transmitted by both Sahih Bukhari and Muslim.

Yet, in spite of all these protective guidelines, the Prophet (SAW), true to the Islamic principle, reminds us that, "No disease is conveyed from the sick to the healthy without Allah's permission."[42] This is also the case in modem medicine because it is not in all cases that persons predisposed to a particular infection acquire the disease. Various factors come into play, which ultimately determine whether a person becomes infected or otherwise. These factors include the immune status of the individual, genetic susceptibility, dose of the inoculation of the pathogenic organism and its virulence and so on and so forth. In truth, all these are natural endowments from Allah. Therefore, the prophetic statements in this regard are in perfect harmony with our present day knowledge of communicable diseases and the methods of preventing them.

2.12   Passing Urine in Stagnant Water

It is also reported from the authority of Abu Hurairah and related in both *Sahah* collections that the Prophet (SAW) said:

> *None amongst you should urinate in standing water and then (take) bath or wash in it.*

It is a historical fact that during the time of the Prophet (SAW) little, if any, was known about the role played by many of the water-borne agents of infection and infestation, particularly their hosts (definitive and intermediate), mode of transmission, life cycles and methods of prevention. It is now known that swimming, bathing, washing or wading in

41. Nasocomial inflection are infections that are transmitted in the hospital environment from patients to other patients or health workers and vice versa.
42. From Abu Hurairah in Sahih Bukhari.

dirty stagnant water carries a high risk of infection with many parasitic or helminthic diseases, such as onchocerciasis, dracunculiasis (guinea worm) and schistosomiasis (bilharziasis), which causes blindness, chronic ulcers, renal failure, cancer of the urinary bladder, liver diseases, pulmonary hypertension, paralysis (paraplegia), brain disorders and death. According to one of the most authoritative texts in the medical sciences:

> *About 5% of the world's population (200 million) is affected by schistosomiasis in about 70 countries, and about 20 million people die (from it) every year.*[43] *In the tropics and subtropics, it is second only to malaria in socio-economic and public health importance.*

Scientific knowledge, much after the prophetic era, on the life cycle of most of these parasites has shown that infestation occurs only when an infected man urinates or defecates into or near fresh water in ponds, puddles, rivers, etc, that the life cycle of the worms is restarted, enabling them to cause hazards to the health of man. This knowledge is now vigorously utilised in designing the strategies or methods of prevention of these infections and infestations.

What is remarkable about the *hadith* above is that, that knowledge, or more precisely the preventive method, was offered to humanity about 1400 years ago from the teachings of an unlettered Arab in the heart of the desert at a time when little, if any, was gathered about water-borne infestations and their mode of transmission or life cycle. In fact, it was not until the development of the microscope by Antony Van Leeuwenhoek in the 17th century, that the microscopic world became visible to the human eye. Even then, it was not until Louis Pasteur's discoveries in the 19th century that science began to understand the relationship between pathogens and diseases.

2.13   Medical Benefits of Ablution and *Salat*

Ablution, which involves spiritual and psychological preparation before commencement of *salat,* is not merely a repetitive process of washing the external parts of the body using pure and uncontaminated water. The medical benefits derivable from the act include; promotion of personal hygiene, aiding peripheral circulation (through the effects of regular massage and body movements), protection from dental carey (mouth rinsing protects and cleans the teeth and gums by removing food remnants and germs) and improvement on general oral hygiene.

It also prevents skin dryness and body odour from continuous mixing of sweat with dirts or dusts on the exposed surface of the body (mainly the distal parts of the limbs). Regular washing and sniffing the nose with water also keeps the nostril clean and moist, thereby preventing epistaxis (nose bleed) arising from the contributory effect of cracking of the thin (mucous) membrane covering the Little's area, especially during the hamattan dry season.

The Little's area is the commonest site of nasal bleeding due to congestion of many blood vessels (plexus) in the anterior end of the nasal septum, its exposure to the outer surface and the inherent weakness or thinness of the membrane covering it.

The *salat,* which does not simply means prayer, comprises both spiritual and physical act that symbolises a communion

---

43. From *Principles and Practice of Surgery including Pathology in the Tropics* by Badoe E.A et al, 2nd Edition, pp.46

between the Worshipped and the worshipper, the Creator and the created.

The Muslims' prayer is a unique form of worship in which the whole body participates by standing, kneeling, sitting and prostrating; the tongue is active with Qur'anic recitation and supplication, the heart is totally engaged in its rhythmic activity, and the mind is occupied by meditation and reflection. As a result of all these, the heart remains active and vigilant with each change of posture or position, supplying oxygenated blood to the skeletal muscles engaged in the physical activity of the *salat* and the repetitive movements of the limbs aids venous (blood) return from the peripheral circulation to the heart. The mind becomes engrossed in co-ordination, activation of memorisation delving into the subconscious while thriving to maintain a balance between the physical and the spiritual, the body and the soul, the here and the hereafter.

Ultimately, the *salat* provides a harmony between the two worlds, a constant reminder of the unity of God, His Supremacy, His Holiness and His absolute Lordship. It is also an appeal to the worshipper, as he or she bow down in prayer to also bow down mentally to carry His Will. The Muslim would then return from the *salat* to the daily occupations of his life with a better emotional, physical and moral state guided by a sound mind with high spirits.

The *salat* among other medical benefits, enhanced blood circulation, promote mental activity and alertness, activates memory and deep reflection. Medical research has also demonstrated its stress-reducing effect on the various organs of the body, possibly through the central and autonomic nervous system. It therefore provides a calming effect on the body, reduces anxiety and lower blood pressure particularly when verses of *Targheeb* (those which foretold glad tidings of the hereafter) are recited.

CHAPTER THREE

Curative Medicine

3.0 Introduction

From the very beginning and not by analogy or extension, the Qur'an announces that it is not only a cure for spiritual malady, but also for physical ones.

> *We reveal of the Qur'an that which is a healing and a mercy to believers (Q17:82).*

> *O mankind, there has come to you an admonition from your Lord and a healing ... (Q10:57).*

> *The issues from within their bodies a drink of varying colours, wherein is healing for men ... (Q16:69).*

In connection with the above verses, it implies that everything which has been revealed in the Qur'an heals. Ali bn Abi Talib (RA) was reported, according to a Tirmidhi transmission, as saying, "The best medicine is the Qur'an." He also said in the same transmission, "The wonders of the Qur'an never cease." The Qur'an, therefore, heals physical disease if it is used for that purpose, just as it cures error, ignorance and doubt. It gives guidance to whoever is lost or bewildered. It cures the body and the mind, the physical and the spiritual, the worldly and the eternal, the seen and the unseen.

Zaid bn Aslam reported in Sahih Muslim that a man was injured in the time of the Prophet (SAW) and blood congealed at the (wounded) spot. The man sent for two men from Bani Ammar. When the two men came, the Apostle of Allah (SAW) asked them, "Which of you knows more medicine?" They said, "Is medicine of any use, O Apostle of Allah?" Zaid said, 'I think the Apostle of Allah declared, "He who has sent the disease also sent the cure." It is also narrated by Abu Hurairah in Sahih Bukhari that the Prophet (SAW) said, "No disease Allah created, apart from old age and death, but that he created its treatment." The Messenger of Allah (SAW) was also reported by Abubakar (RA) in Sahih Muslim saying, "Every disease has a cure. Knowing the right medicine will cure the disease by God's leave."

In a *hadith* which has been transmitted by Abu Na'im (RA), Hassan Thn Urwah said, "I never met anyone who knew more about medicine than Aisha (RA), the wife of the Prophet (SAW). I once said to her, "I am astonished by your insight into medicine, O Mother of the Faithful", and she answered, "O son of my sister, whenever any member of my family was ill, the Prophet used to prescribe a remedy for them. So I used to remember it, and then prescribe the same for other people."

Since the time of its revelation, the Qur'an has been used by the Prophet (SAW) and many of his *Sahaba* (companions) as a direct healing modality in many ways. Such ways involve:

- The recitation of the Qur'an and supplication to God for healing (this is the spiritual medicine).

- The usage of suggested therapeutic agents by the Qur'an.

For example, honey (this is the natural medicine).

• The combination of spiritual and natural medicine.

The noble Prophet (SAW) endowed with great knowledge and making use of his great logical and scientific mind, made certain pronouncements and carried out specific procedures meant to provide a healing effect on disease and injuries. The Qur'an and Sunnah thus provide guidance on natural and spiritual medicine in treating many diseases. Some of these methodologies will be analysed briefly.

3.1 Treatment with Honey

The Qur'an states:

> And your Lord taught the Bee to build its cells in hills from within, on trees and, in (men's) habitations. Then to eat of all the produce (of the earth). And follow the Ways of your Lord made smooth: there issues from within their bodies a drink of varying colours, wherein is healing for men: Verily in this is a sign for those who give thought (Q16:68-69).

It is narrated by Abu Sa'id AI-Khudri in the *Sahah* transmissions, that:

> *A man came to God's Prophet (SAW) and reported that his brother was complaining of irregular bowel movement. Allah's Messenger (SAW) advised, "Make him drink honey". The man came back and said, "I made him take honey but it did not help!" The Messenger of Allah (SAW) gave the same advise for two or three times, and the man kept coming back with the*

same answer. After the third or the fourth time, Allah's Messenger (SAW) then said, God spoke the truth, and your brother's abdomen has told a lie. And he made the man to drink it (honey) and he was cured.

It should be noted from the *hadith* how an inadequate intake of several doses of the drug (honey) were not effective enough to provide a cure to the man's ailment until the last dose was taken. The successive commands of the Prophet (SAW) may very likely be an emphasis on the dosage regime - which is an extension of the Prophet's idea and concept of "knowing the right medicine will cure the disease." We also highlight that the emphasis of the Prophet on patience and perseverance to a sick person, may be a pointer to the mechanism of diseases and drugs, for it is not all of a sudden that a man recovers from a disease whether it is treated or untreated, because in most cases it entails a series of events that may ultimately lead to a complete recovery.

Aisha (RA), the wife of the Prophet (SAW), used to recommend *At- Talbina* (a kind of porridge prepared from honey, milk and white barley flour) for the treatment of the sick. She used to say, "I heard Allah's Messenger saying, "*At-Talbina* gives rest to the heart of the patient and makes it active and relieves some of his sorrow or grief."[44]

It is transmitted in Sahih Muslim that Abu Hurairah narrated in the *hadith* that the Prophet (SAW) said, "Whosoever eats honey (at least) three times every month will meet with no great affliction." In another tradition narrated from Thn Mas 'ud in Mishkat, God's Messenger (SAW) said, "Make use of the two remedies; honey and the Qur' an."

---

44. Bukhari and Muslim transmission.

In this saying, the Prophet (SAW) has linked human and divine medicine, remedies for the body and those of the soul, the natural and the spiritual factor and the earthly medicine and the heavenly one.

Ibn Juray said, "I heard Al-Zuhri saying, "Resort to honey as it is conducive to the activation of memorisation." Imam Ibn Qayyim (the famous scholar and disciple of Ibn Taimiyyah) in his *Tibbi Nabawi* (The Prophetic Medicine) said about honey:

> *Honey is an abluent and an aperient. It contains detergent and tonic properties that cleanse the arteries and the bowels of impurities, opens obstructions of the liver, kidney and blad-der. Honey is superior to sugar in many respects, and it is less sweet but stronger, and if taken excessively, can be harmful to the bile, unless it is mixed with vinegar. Honey is good for the aged, it is a cough suppressant and is also a curative for a depraved appetite, and when taken as a drink mixed with hot water and a pomade made from sweet roses, it helps the treat-ment of rabies, and is considered a safeguard against further infections. Honey is also used as a detoxification agent for drug users and as an antitoxin to treat plant poison. As a preservative, honey can be used to preserve meat for up to three months, and various kind of fruits for up to six months. Known as 'the trustworthy preservative', honey was used as a principal ingredient in embalming the dead.[45] Spreading natural raw honey over one's hair as ointment will cure head lice and other parasites. It also promotes hair growth. Honey brightens the*

*vision and when used as a mouth wash, it
whitens the teeth, strengthens the gums and
eliminates gum diseases. Honey indeed has a
great nutritional value and is the drink of
drinks, a sweetener of sweeteners, an ointment
of ointments, and there is no other food among
what God Al-mighty has created for us that
equals honey in value, and nothing is close to
its constitution.*

From the above and many other related *hadith,* it is clear
that the holy Prophet and his companions and the generation
of Muslim scholars after them had used honey in the
treatment of many diseases, such as abdominal discomfort,
diarrhoea, heart diseases, wound healing, respiratory tract
infections, endocrine disorders and so on.

The medicinal values of honey are indeed remarkable.
In fact, it is a cure for many kinds of diseases. It is scientifically
known that honey contains almost all the food molecules
that aid growth and energy utilisation. It contains many
amino acids, vitamins, carbohydrates and other essential
elements. It provides the body with a rich supply of amino
acids, which aid the defense against infection, the
regeneration of cells and body repair from injury. The
nutritive value of honey was clearly demonstrated by several
medical researches conducted on newborn infants and
children with muscular atrophy and severe chronic
nutritional disturbances. Prior to these, a scientific research
conducted in 1974 at Tamagawa University in Japan, showed
that the amino acid content of honey is the same as that
found in human, cow and goat milk (however, the proportion
for each differs), hence confirming that honey is of higher

---

45. The early Egyptian Physicians used honey in the mummification of
     dead bodies.

nutritional value. Apart from other uses, honey is strongly recommended in the treatment of wounds from burns (or scalds), abscesses, dehiscence, traumatic injury, cancers and varieties of ulcers, etc. According to one of the most authoritative texts in surgical practice:

> *Honey applied daily (to a wound) is effective in preventing bacterial contamination and in promoting healing.*[46]

The scientific basis for the use of honey in wound management and a variety of ulcers depends on its intrinsic value or constitution. Pure natural honey is non-allergenic, non-toxic and non-adherent to tissues, and is completely sterile (unless contaminated) and therefore provides a good dressing material that can prevent secondary wound infection or sepsis. Honey has an acidic PH of about 4.5, which does not favour bacterial growth and survival. Being highly hydrophilic; honey dehydrates any living bacteria within its vicinity. In addition, honey is found to contain substances which are directly or indirectly lethal to bacteria by reacting with tissue peroxidases to release oxygen free radicals, which are toxic to bacteria.

Research has also shown that honey contains a substance called *inhibin,* a heat liable antibiotic to which many bacteria are sensitive. Apart from its antimicrobial agents, the nutritive elements in it provide nutrients to the healing tissues and encourage the formation and growth of granulation tissue. Following a research work conducted at the Lagos University Teaching Hospital, Nigeria, to "re-examine the claim that honey used alone is effective in healing wounds at various sites and disease entities," it was observed that:

---

46. See Badoe E.A et al (1994): *Principles and Practice of Surgery including Pathology in the Tropics,* (2nd ed.).

> *Weeping wounds dried up, necrotic wounds sloughed off, leaving healthy granulating tissues and malodorous wounds stop being so following a few days of honey treatment.* [47]

It is interesting to note that before the commencement of honey treatment, a bacteriological study was conducted from wound cultures and an antibiotic sensitivity test was also carried out. The findings showed that the wound cultures yielded organisms such as *Klebsiella aerogenes, Proteus mirabilis, Escherichia coli, Pseudomonas aeruginosa, Streptococcus pyogenes* and *Staphylococci,* but after one week of honey dressing, no single organism was cultured from the wound and 100% treatment success was therefore achieved. The fact that antibiotic sensitivity spectrum showed that some of the organisms were sensitive to antibiotics (such as streptomycin, colistin, tetracycline, ampicillin, cloxacillin, erythromycin, sulphadiazine, etc), implies that by extension, honey has the potential to provide a potent substitute for all these antibiotics.[48]

Of recent, a further scientific research on honey conducted by researchers and scientists in the United States of America has led to the production of different preparations of honey extracts into several drug formulations (one of which is marketed as Roy gel ultima or Royal jelly). This royal jelly is a complex substance secreted by the salivary glands of the honey bee (the worker or "nurse" bee in particular). The duty of the young worker bee is to nourish the larvae with the royal jelly through which they obtain rapid growth and full development to become the future queen bees. Of all the

---

47. See "Effect of Natural Honey on Wound Management – A pilot Study" by Atimomo C.E. Ohwovoriole A.E and Anyiwo C.E. in *The Nigerian Medical Practitioner* Vol.20.No.2 1996, pp. 23-35.

female bees, therefore, only the queen bees are fertile and sexually developed (each producing some 400,000 eggs annually).[49]

Although the 20-30,000 worker bees and several hundred drones (in the hive) live for only a few months, remarkably the queen bee live as long as six (6) years! Thus, scientists engage in the research are of the opinion that a constituent of the honey (precisely the royal jelly), which the worker bees feed the queen, might have something to do with increasing the life span of these insects and maintaining their sound health.

At the medical congress held in Karisruhe, Germany, the general consensus of scientists who have performed research on honey was that, it was found to be an excellent tonic for the nerves, provides a feeling of well being, relieves depression and anxiety, restores natural vitality and gives a more youthful disposition in the patient. In both men and women,

48. Spectacular as the research was, it represent a continuity or extension of works done by several scientists in different parts of the world, who confirmed the confirmed the efficacy of honey in enhancing the healing of wounds and ulcers.
49. In the honey bee colony, the queen is solely responsible for laying eggs, the drones for fertilizing the queen, while the workers gather food and perform sundry duties in the hive. Each caste is adapted for its particular job; thus the queen is a fertile female, the drones fertile males and the workers sterile females with well developed mouthpart and other structural adaptation for collecting nectar and pollen. When the queen lays eggs, some are fertilized and some are not.

The unfertilised (haploid) eggs develop into males (drones) and the fertilized (diploid) eggs develop into female (queen or workers). Whether a female bee becomes a queen or a worker depend on its diet and again, the particular diet they feed upon determine their structural modification, job adaptation and longevity or life spain! If a Larva is fed on nothing but the royal jelly, a queen eventually emerges from a pupa and live as long as six (6) years. If, however the royal jelly is replaced after few days by a different diet, a worker or drone emerges from the pupae and live an average of only five (5) months!

honey is known to improve memory, rejuvenate sexual capacities and help alleviate some of the medical problems of senility (old age). Researchers have attributed honey's potency to vitamins and hormones. Dr Fredirick Banting, the discoverer of insulin, has suggested pantothenic acid. But the most recent opinion is that honey's stimulating qualities will eventually be attributed to a "natural X factor," which cannot be produced synthetically.

Honey is also known to be a gland activator. It increases the activity of the pituitary, thyroid, adrenal cortex and the pancreatic glands. Scientific reports have confirmed that honey helps patients suffering from atherosclerosis, gingivitis, stomatitis, various skin disorders, alopecia, circulatory disturbances and rheumatoid arthritis.

Hence, from such extensive healing traits among other properties in this divine gift, we can understand the meaning contained in the Qur'anic verse:

And she has been given everything (Q27:23).

3.2   Fever, Sore 'Throat and Tonsilitis

Concerning the affliction of Prophet Job (AS), the Qur'an states:

> *Behold he cried to his Lord: 'Satan has afflicted me with dis-tress and suffering!' (We said): "Strike with your foot, here is water wherein to wash, cool and refreshing, and to drink." (Q38:41-42).*

Commentators of the revised Abdullahi Yusuf Ali translation of the holy Qur'an, said on this verse, "Prophet Job (AS) was afflicted with loathsome sores and material distress for which he was commanded to strike the earth with his foot, and a fountain gushed forth to give him a bath, refresh his spirit and to give him drink and rest, and the recuperative process begun."

It is reported from Aisha (RA), the wife of the Prophet and Abdullahi Ibn Umar in the *Sahah* transmissions, that the Messenger of Allah (SAW) said:

> *Fever is from the heat of hell, so cool it with water.*

It is also narrated from Fatima bint Mundhir that whenever a woman suffering from fever came to Asma'u bint Abubakar, she would send for water and poured it on her and would say that:

> *The Apostle of Allah used to order the cooling of fever by means of water.*

Compare this procedure with our present day "tepid sponging" in the management or control of fever, especially in children. There are many other narrations in which the Prophet treated fever with a water bath, advising his companions to do the same.

Concerning the treatment of tonsilitis, Ummi Qaisi, daughter of Mihsan, narrated in the *Sahah* collections as follows:

> *I visited Allah's Apostle (SAW) along with my son (who had not been weaned) whose palate and tonsils I had pressed with my finger as a treatment for disease.*

The Prophet (SAW) said, "Why do you pain your children by pressing their throats! Use *ud-al Hindi* (leaves from the Indian aloe tree mixed with oils) for it cures seven diseases, one of which is tonsilitis." [50]

3.3 The Control of Bleeding and the Treatment of Wounds

Sahal bn Sa' ad narrated that:

> *On the day of the battle of Uhud, God's Messenger (SAW) was wounded in the face, his eyetooth (incisor) broke, and his helmet collapsed over his head. I saw his daughter Fatima (RA) cleaning his wound and steadily wiping the blood flowing allover his face. I also saw Ali (RA) standing at her side and using his armour as a basin to wash the wound with water. When she realized that she could not control the bleeding, she cut off a small piece of straw mat made of papyrus, burned it to ashes and applied it to his wound whereupon the bleeding stopped.*

The prime message to note here is the cleaning of the wound with water and the application of a "sterilised" material (that is, by burning it, which is a routine procedure even in modem microbiology laboratories) and also the choice of the papyrus tree. In fact, ashes produced from papyrus strains have been reported by scholars to possess strong agglutinating effects for clumping together the blood cells and in suspending the flow of blood (shunting). Such ashes are also highly absorbent and less irritating for wounds. Using dry papyrus ashes as powder or mixing it with vinegar can

---

50. The original word used in the translation was pleurisy, I consider tonsillitis to be more appropriate in view of the specifications made to palate and tonsils and other corroborating *ahadith* which made mention of pressing the uvula, the inflammation of the throat and *uthra* as "an ulcer that originates in an inflammation between the ear and the throat, and mostly affects children." Allah knows best.

stop epistaxis or nose bleeding *(ruaj)*. In his famous book, *The Canon of Medicine*, Ibn Sina also mentioned its use as an antiseptic agent to sterilise fresh wounds, clot the blood and also prevent the spread of malignant ulcerations.

3.4 Cupping and Cauterisation

Ibn Abbas and J abir narrated in the *Sahah* collections that Allah's Apostle (SAW) said:

> *Healing is in three things, a gulp of honey, cupping and cauterisation, but I do not like to be cauterised.*

Cupping is a method of counter-irritation whereby an animal horn is applied to the skin with a resultant suction producing hyperaemia or drawing clotted blood to the surface (blood-letting). Usually the skin is scarified before placing the cup or horn. Cupping as a curative procedure is meant to dry out internal inflammation and remove "bad" blood from the body. It is also said to be helpful for a woman with abnormal amenorrhoea in provoking her menstrual flows.

Whatever cupping entails and the claims associated with it, our present day cupping is in the form of exchange blood transfusion and auto-transfusion and the like. Exchange blood transfusion involves the replacement of a patient's blood by donor blood, performed by repeated withdrawal of the recipient's "bad" blood and the transfusion of donor's "good" blood until most of the patient's blood has been replaced. This procedure is used mainly in the treatment of babies with Rhesus incompatibility isoimmune haemolytic anaemia (erythro-blastosis foetalis), hyperbiluribinaemia (mainly unconjugated) and septicaemia. In the case of auto-transfusion (also called auto-reinfusion), the procedure involves the transfusion of blood into the subject from whom it has been obtained or from whom it has escaped, as from internal haemorrhage.

Furthermore, it should be understood that there are certain medical practices which predated the advent of the Prophet (SAW), which he either encouraged, discouraged or left unchanged. Cupping is one such method that was existent in Arabia even before the coming of the Prophet, and which he left untouched due to the needs of the time and the limitations imposed by the given circumstances. Thus, in this light we can understand the logic of advising people to rely on simple practices, such as cupping, at a time when there were limited possibilities for the scientific use of drugs. Moreover, in the light of the prophesy of Allah's Messenger (SAW) that, "he who lives long among you would see a great deal of changes on certain things" and the remarkable advances in modern medicine, cupping has no place in present day clinical practice.[51]

Though the above can be said of cupping, it cannot in the case of scarification, which is part of the clinical procedure prior to cupping. For long, it has been known that scarification, as a form of mechanical stimulation of the skin, can be used to provide relief from pain. It has been scientifically established that pain transmission to the high centres of the brain can be inhibited or blocked by simple manoeuvres such as rubbing or scarifying the skin. The same principle also explains acupuncture, an oriental method of treating pain and disease or producing surgical anaesthesia. The neural mechanism for this blockade or antagonism has

---

51. It is associated with a lot of complication such as haemorrhage, hypovolaemic shock, thromboembolism, air embolisim, anaemia, disseminated intravascular coagulopathy, denervation, scar or kel-oid formation and the transmission of infection to the person being cupped, as well as the cupper and so on.

been partly explained by the gate control theory and the stimulation of naturally existing brain peptides with analgesic properties.

With regards to cauterisation, this is a procedure of causing the destruction of tissues by applying a heated instrument, a usually sharp iron rod or metal. Cauterisation is an emergency method of treatment permitted only under dire need just as in the case with amputation. Moreover, cauterisation is discouraged by the Prophet (SAW). Thus, the Apostle of Allah (SAW) favoured the use of honey and gave precedence of cupping over cauterisation. In another prophetic tradition, the Messenger of God (SAW) said, "I personally do not like to use cauterization."

Thus, it is only when all other remedies have failed, that one is allowed to try cautery. According to Imam As-Suyuti, it should only be used when the strongest medicine has been defeated by the body constitution and no other remedy has proved successful or is nowhere available. It is reported by Jabir in a Sahib Muslim transmission, that the Apostle of Allah sent a physician to Ubay bn Ka'b (who sustained an arrow injury on the medial vein of his arm). He (the Physician) cut the vein and then cauterised it. With regards to the *hadith* in which the Prophet (SAW) himself cauterised Sa' ad, AI-Khattabi said, "Truly the Prophet cauterised Sa' ad in order to stop haemorrhage, which otherwise would have been fatal." Hence, cauterisation is also practised after the amputation of a hand or foot as a matter of obligation. In his *Tibbi Nabawi*, As-Suyuti even went as far as explaining the mechanism of cauterisation:

> *Cauterisation is fully permitted whenever there is no alternative – for example, where a wound has pierced an artery and the bleeding would not stop normally unless it is cauterised with fire. This is because the pumping in the artery*

> *prevents the blood from clotting. But with cauterisation, a scab is formed at the mouth of the wound, so that the blood which is flowing from the puncture in the artery can cling to it at the mouth of the wound and clotting takes place.*

It should be noted that the use of diathermy in modern surgical practice is a modification and improvement upon cauterisation by fire. Diathermy involves the passage of an electric current through tissues, commonly used to stop bleeding by the coagulation of blood, or to cut through tissues during surgical operations. Diathermy was first used in modem surgery in 1910 and today after it has undergone tremendous development, it remains one of the most valuable facilities in the operating theatre, occupying a prominent position in the armamentarium of the modem day surgeon.

> *What cannot be cured with medicaments is cured by the knife, what the knife cannot cure is cured with the searing iron, and whatever this cannot cure must be considered incurable.*
> – Hippocrates in *The Book of Aphorism.*

3.5 Remedy with Dates

The Qur'an states:

> *And shake towards thyself the trunk of the palm tree. It will let fall fresh ripe dates upon thee. So eat and drink and cool (thine) eyes (Q19:25-26). And tall (and stately) palm-trees, with shoots of fruit-stalks, piled one over another; as sustenance for Allah's servants (Q50:10-11).*

Mujahid narrated in Sunan Abu Dawud that Sa'id (RA) said:

> *The Messenger of Allah (SAW) visited me during a sickness I had; he placed his hands between my nipples, and I felt its cooling blessings in the organs that lie within the chest wall.*
> *He then commented, 'You are suffering from the enlargement of the heart. Call for Al-Harith bn Kaladah. He practises medicine. Ask him to take seven dried dates (ajwa), crush them with their seeds to form a medicinal compound, and let him massage your chest with their paste.'*

Sa'ad bn Abi Waqqas (RA) reported in the Sahib Bukhari and the Muslim transmission that he heard Allah's Apostle saying, "If somebody takes seven *ajwa* dates every morning, he will not be affected by poison or magic that day." In Sunan of an-Nasa'i and Majah, two *hadith* were reported from the authority of Jabir and Abi Sa'id (RA) that Allah's Messenger (SAW) said, "The pressed dates are derived from heaven and provide a cure against poison and their water palliates ocular harms."[52] In another *hadith* from Abu Hurairah, the Prophet (SAW) also said, "In the sweetness of *al·Bumiy* dates, there is no disease."

From the above *hadith*, the Prophet (SAW) not only pinpoints the medicinal benefits of dates but also specifies their types or categories (For example, *Ajwa, al·Bumiy, Ratib, Balah, Tamr,* etc), thereby leaving us with the challenge to conduct research on their chemical constitution and benefits. We can also deduce from the *hadith* that the Prophet (SAW)

---

52. Meaning eye problems.

also recommended dates as a prophylaxis against many diseases such as food poisoning and blindness. Scientifically, dates are known to be rich in minerals and vitamins (A, B and D), protein, sugar and gelatin. Thus, their relevance in preventing blindness is indeed great.

It has been medically established that vitamin A plays an important role in the maintenance of the integrity of the epithelial tissues, synthesis of mucopolysaccharides (collagen synthesis, growth of long bones and connective tissues), maintaining the stability of cell membranes and the formation of the visual pigment (rhodopsin and iodopsin), which promotes eye sight. According to Emeritus Professor of oral medicine and pathology, Roderick Cawson and his colleagues:

> *Vitamin A is a fat soluble factor and the best known effect of its deficiency is the inability to see in weak light (night blindness). One of the earliest effect of Vitamin A deficiency is the impairment of the formation of visual pigments, with the result that vision in poor light deteriorates and later degenerative changes develop in the retina.* [53]

3.6   Remedy with Nigella Seed *(Habba-tus-Sawda)*

Abu Hurairah and Aisha (RA) narrated in the *Sahah* collections that God's Messenger said:

> *Use this black seed regularly, because it has a cure for every disease except cancer and that is a fatal disease.*[54]

---

53. The most sensitive and delicate layer of the eye that mediate vision.
54. In another narration, it reads: "Use this black seed regularly because it has a cure for every disease except death."

The black seed *(Habba-tu Sawda*[55]*)* is the common fennel flower of the plant *(Nigella Sativa)*. A special oil is extracted from the seeds which is then used in the preparation of medical formulas. Scholars in prophetic medicine said that the seed can be used in the treatment of many diseases, such as bronchitis, cough and the common cold. It is also said to increase body tone, act as a digestive tonic, quell belching, stimulate the excretion of urine, quell colic pain, de-worm the gastro-intestinal tract, remove patches of leucoderma, benefit some skin allergies, treat fever, open obstructions, stimulate menstrual period, increase the flow of breast milk and has a calming effect on the nervous and respiratory systems.

Therefore, it is helpful in treating pertussis, dry cough, asthma and bronchial respiratory complaints. It causes irritation of the digestive system when taken unmixed or undiluted, acting as a purgative. This is the *Habba-tu s-Sawdal* But that is not all. In his *Canon of Medicine,* Thn Sina maintains that, "The black seed acts as an expectorant, it stimulates the body's energy and helps recovery from fatigue and dispiritedness."

The black seed is known to reduce swellings and remove scales in ringworm. Drinking a decoction of crushed black seeds mixed with honey is said to dissolve gall stones and kidney stones, and when taken over a few days it increases the rate of flow of urine, menses and milk. An ointment of black seeds also stimulates the growth of the beard and can prevent hair graying. It also claims usefulness in the treatment of jaundice, headache; the common cold, nasal congestion, facial paralysis, tetanus, and haemorrhoids. As a fumigant, the smoke of *Habba tus-Sawda* drives away flying

---

55. Also called Black cumin, Coriander seeds, Indian cumin, Blessed seed *(Habbatul Baraka)*, Arabian seed (because of its habitat), etc.

insects. In fact, the medicinal benefits contained in the black seeds are numerous.

Concerning *Habbatus-Sawda*, several medical benefits have been ascribed to it, some of which have been confirmed through practical life experience and empirical deductions, but a greater part of its benefits remains unknown or unsubstantiated due to lack of adequate research on the drug. In Al-Alkili's translation of Ibn Qayyim's *Tibbi Nabawi*, a reference was made to a publication on *habbatus-sawda*, which appeared in the Egyptian Pharmaceutical Bulletin titled, "Some Chemical and Pharmacological Properties of the New Drug *Nigellone.*" It is said that some pharmaceutical industries in the Middle East are currently conducting research on the drug and have even reached the stage of clinical trials using different formulations (ointments, emulsions, powder, etc). Whatever the case, presently adequate information about the drug is not conventionally available. Thus, the challenge remains ours.

From the little work done so far on *habbatu-sawda*, it is suggested that its therapeutic effect lies in the potency of a special oil extracted from its seed, and that the oil contains elements such as ketone and thiamine, which are constituents of normal body requirement.

3.7 Diseases of and Antidotes to the Housefly

Abu Hurairah (RA) narrated in Sahih Bukhari that the Messenger of Allah (SAW) said:

> *If a fly falls in the vessel of anyone of you let him dip all of it (into the vessel) and throw it away, for in one of its wings there is a disease and in the other (wing) there is healing (antidote for it) for the disease.*

Medically, it is well known that the fly carries some pathogens in some parts of its body, as mentioned by the Prophet (SAW) about 1400 years ago when humanity knows very little of medicine. It is a scientific fact that some organisms contain some chemicals (secretions) which when released kill the offending organism or pathogens. For example, the naturally occurring penicillin (such as *penicillin G or benzyl penicillin*), which kills pathogenic organisms like staphylococci, clostridia, etc, is derived from fungal molds - *Penicillin no tatum*. Conversely, some bacteria release an enzyme - penicillinase, which inactivates penicillin by hydrolysing the *lactam bond* (an important factor in the resistance against infection). Moreover, microbiologists have proved that there are longitudinal yeast cells living as parasites inside the belly of the fly,[56] which proliferate through the respiratory tubule of the fly. If the fly is dipped in a liquid, these cells burst in the fluid to release chemical substances which act as an antidote for the pathogens which the fly carries.

3.8 Remedy with Milk

The Qur' an states:

> *And verily in cattle (too) will you find instructive signs from what is within their bodies, between excretions and blood, We produce for your drink milk, pure and agreeable to those who drink it (Q16:66).*

It is reported from the authority of Ibn Abbas (RA) in Abu Da' wud and Tirmidhi transmissions that the Prophet (SAW) said:

---

56. Of the species *Musca domestica* (common housefly) or *Fannia canicularis* (lesser housefly).

> *Let whosoever is given milk by Allah say, 'May the blessing of Allah be in it, and may He give us more of it' , for I know that there is no other food or drink that can take its place.*

In another *hadith*, the Prophet (SAW) also said, "Drink *Laban* (cow's milk), for it is a healing and fattening remedy", According to Ibn Mas'ud (RA), the Prophet added "". for the cow feed on all sorts of plants."

Scientifically, it is known that milk is a rich source of proteins, minerals and certain trace elements, and thus aids body growth and development. Of all other types of milk from animals, *Laban* (cow's milk), as specified by the Prophet (SAW), has the singular and unique quality of being close to the human (breast) milk in constitution in terms of proteins, amino acids, certain carbohydrates and antibodies (which act against the agents of infection). Milk, therefore, is clinically used in the management of malnutrition (particularly in children), peptic ulcer diseases, dyspepsia, constipation, food or chemical poisoning (For example, kerosine), etc. It is also used as part of the special diet for patients with metabolic diseases, such as diabetes mellitus and in nutritional support or therapy for pre-operative and post-operative patients.

3.9   The Treatment of Pain and Malaise

Uthman bn Abu Al-As narrated that he went to the Apostle of Allah (SAW) and complained about some chronic pain he suffered. The Prophet (SAW) said, "Pass your hand seven times upon the seat of pain and say, 'I seek refuge in the honour and power of Allah from the evil that has come upon me' Uthman said, "I recited accordingly and my pain vanished." In another *hadith* Aisha (RA) narrated that whenever the Messenger of Allah (SAW) paid a visit to a patient or a patient was brought to him he used to invoke Allah saying:

> *O Lord and Cherisher of human beings, relieve these sufferings and cure this servant. Indeed, You alone has the power of healing, and You alone can effect permanent recovery.* [57]

This *ruqya* prayer embodies the glorification of His oneness *(Tawheed)*, the cognisance *(Ihsan)* of His knowledge of everything and the acknowledgment of His absolute Lordship *(rububiyya)*.

3.10 The Management of the Unconscious Patient

The Qur'an states concerning the companions of the cave *(As-habul Kahfi)*:

> *We drew (a veil) over their ears, for a number of years, in the cave, so that they heard not. You would have thought them awake, while they were asleep, and we turn them on their right hand and on their left sides (Q18:11 and 18).*

The care of the unconscious patient occupies a special place in clinical medicine. It is an essential requirement that the patient receives a well monitored nursing care that is oriented and geared towards the maintenance of clear airways, the prevention of pressure sores or ulcers, muscle contractures, paraparesis or paralysis, urolithiasis (stones in

---

57. From Sahih Bukhari and Muslim.

the urinary tracts), urinary tract infections and skin diseases among others.

The majority of these complications (of immobilisation) can be avoided and prevented by simply turning the patient regularly from side to side – a form of physiotherapy.

The verses quoted above constitute part of the Qur'anic account of the companions of the cave, that is, *As-habul Kahfi*, who were youth "who believed in their Lord" and were persecuted, so they left the town and hid themselves in a cave in a mountain nearby. It was there in the cave that God rendered them unconscious – "sealed their ears" with their knowledge and ideas remaining at the point in time when they had entered the cave. They were said to be in that state of coma or "sleep" for about three hundred (300) years and when they awoke to consciousness, they had lost all account of time. Here again, God Almighty demonstrated further His signs and power, a lesson for the entire humanity - lessons which are morally, spiritually, physically and medically inclined.

On the medical aspect of the lessons of these verses, the following are noteworthy:[58]

- The verse clearly distinguishes between life and death and that the state of unconsciousness lies somewhere midway.

- That an unconscious patient has no orientation of time, place, persons or things.

---

58. During the review of this work, our attention was drawn to the medical aspect of the story of the companions of the cave by our dedicated and meticulous brother and superior colleague, Dr I.A. Mungadi (Consultant of General Surgery, Usmanu Danfodiyo University Teaching Hospital Sokoto, Nigeria). He also related some Qur'anic verses with the medical concept of the management of burns and dehydration. May Allah bless our scientists and scholars for their commitment to *Ijtihad* for the progress of the Ummah.

- That it is an essential requirement to offer special nursing care to an unconscious patient to prevent the development of the complications of immobilisation.

- That normal body metabolism requires a certain degree of temperature for it to be sustained. Hence, the strategic position they occupied in relation to sunlight, ensures that their metabolic processes were not totally arrested.

  > *You would have seen the sun, when it rose, declining to the right from their cave, and when it sets, turning from them to the left, while they lay in the open space in the midst of the cave. Such are among the signs of Allah (Q18: 17).*

- That the sun turning away from them on either sides provide a cooling effect that seemed to cause metabolic inhibition for the preservation of their bodies for a long period.

- That the entire condition suggests that though they were asleep, their biological functions were inhibited (intermittently) to avoid the usual demands of a normal metabolic processes (water and food requirement, excretory needs, etc)

- That the verse, 'you would have thought them awake, while they were asleep' suggests that their eyes were blinking. Otherwise, prolong closure of the eye will lead to blindness resulting from optic atrophy and conversely prolonged eye opening will also lead to blindness arising from corneo-xerosis. Consequently, the Qur'an describes this amazingly as an usual state that will cause an observer to be 'filled with terror'.

3.11 The Management of Burns and Dehydration

The Qur'an states:

> The companions of the fire will call to the companions of the Garden: "Pour down to us water or anything that Allah doth provide for your sustenance" (Q7:50).

It has been related from the authority of Thn Umar and Thn Abbas (RA) that the Messenger of Allah (SAW) said:

> Fever is from the raging heat of the fire, so cool it down with water.[59]

Burns are among the most serious and feared injuries that can afflict humankind (no wonder holy scriptures specify them as the ultimate punishment for wrongdoers). Most of the pathologic processes initiated by burns are inflammatory in nature and manifest among other things with desquamation of the skin, vesicles (blisters), necrosis of the dermis and epidermis and the neuro-vascular supply of the area. A variety of systemic effects also complicate certain bums, leading to a wide range of metabolic responses proportionate to the degree of injury. The most serious problems following severe burns are the consequences of dehydration, particularly hypovolaemic shock, which is fatal and can lead to death within the first twenty-four hours.

Thus, in the management of burns, fluid replacement (after resuscitation) is the single, most important factor in combating immediate life-threatening complications, such as hypovolaemic shock, renal failure, septicaemia (infection) and anaemia. From the verse also, emphasis is laid on nutritional support or therapy – "give us water or anything

---

59. This *hadith* was transmitted by both Sahih Bukhari and Muslim.

for sustenance," which is an important factor in wound healing, tissue growth and body repair from injury. Another verse of the Qur'an states:

> Those who reject Our signs, We shall soon cast (them) into the fire: as often as their skins are roasted through. We shall change them for fresh skins, that they may taste the chastisement, for Allah is exalted in power, Wise (Q4:56).

With regards to the above, Muslim scholars and scientists are of the opinion that the verse is a pointer to the scientific fact that, the skin contains nerve endings or pain receptors that are responsible for pain transmission. Hence, the creation of a "fresh skin" for repetitive pain stimulation as a punishment signifies Allah's wisdom and knowledge concerning every detail of the human body and of other created beings.

3.12 Nutritional Rehabilitation in Patients' Care

The Qur'an states:

> O you Messengers!, eat (all) things good and pure, and work righteousness (Q23:51).

Concerning Mary, the mother of Jesus (AS), who was assigned to the care of Prophet Zachariah [Zakariyya (AS)], the Qur'an states:

> Every time that he entered (her chamber) to see her, he found her supplied with sustenance ... for Allah provides sustenance to whom He pleases without measure (Q3:37).

It has been related by Aisha (RA) from Allah's Messenger (SAW) that, "Whenever any of the companions of the Prophet (SAW) were sick, he would order a soup to be made for them, and he would make them drink the soup. He used to say that, "It would comfort the innermost parts of the sick, wiping away affliction and sickness just as dust is wiped away from the face."[60] Ibn Abbas (RA) also reported the Messenger of Allah (SAW) as saying, "If any of you is sick, and he has an appetite for something, then he should eat it."[61]

3.13 The Treatment of Mental Illnesses and Other Diseases

The Qur'an states:

> *(Evil ones) among men and Jions inspiring each other with flowery discourses by way of deception (Q6: 112).*

Again:

> *Say: I seek refuge with the Lord and Cherisher of mankind, ... From the mischief of the whisperer (of evil) who withdraws (after his whisper), among Jions and among men (Q114:1-5).*

Spiritual remedies are the real antidote against necromancy, witchery, the evil eye, psychosomatic and psychiatric disorders. As regards all these, the Prophet (SAW) recommended the regular recitation of the two guardian chapters - *Suratul Falaq* and *Naas* (113 and 114), the Opening

---

60. Tirmidhi transmission.
61. Ibn Majah transmission.

chapter - *Suratul F atiha* (l) and the verse of the divine throne - *Ayatul-Kursiyyu* (2: 255). Besides these Qur'anic verses, there are also special prayers recommended by the Messenger of Allah (SAW).

The *Ruqya* treatment of diseases sometimes will involve exorcism, that is, driving out an evil spirit by prayers. This is one area where divine medicine differs from modern medicine. However, comparing the extent of scientific knowledge to the divine revelations *(wahayi)* Allah, the Almighty, inspired His Messenger (SAW) concerning what benefits man or what may harm him, is like comparing the extent of the total of scientific discoveries to date to the infinite knowledge contained in the universe. In fact, the knowledge God's Messengers (PBUT) possessed cannot be fully measured even by the most ingenious of physicians and scientists with their most sophisticated instruments! Even today a trained medical doctor may feel illiterate or ignorant in comparison with the power of the divine healer, such a physician becomes like the village old woman who prescribes chicken soup for a case of fever!

As for the treatment of people possessed by evil spirits, it is totally an aspect of spiritual medicine. The success or otherwise of this treatment also depends on the skill, faith, purity, prayers and the strong spirit of the exorcist, otherwise his interference will be of no benefit and may even be dangerous for both the patient and the doctor. In the case of a true Sheikh, [62] it may even be sufficient for him to banish such an alien spirit by directly addressing it and firmly saying to it: *Ukhrij minhu* - Get out of him, or he can invoke the

---

62. A well learned and pious Muslim scholar. The term is also used to refer to an aged person and the two meanings may be applied implicitly based on the common observation that acquisition of vast knowledge correlates with advancement in age. The word is analogous to the word Professor in an academic environment.

power of God's name upon it. It is narrated in the traditions that God's Messenger (SAW) used to address such spirits by saying, "Get out of him, O enemy of Allah. I am the Messenger of Allah, and I command you to do so." [63]

Sometimes, the alien spirit may be a rebel demon *(marid)*, who will only come out of the patient by force. From the traditions, *ruqya* is also used in the palliative treatment of various kinds of illnesses, such as pains, boils, anxiety and sorrow, suppurations, cuts, etc. [64]

3.14 The Treatment of Insomnia or Sleep Disorder

The Qur'an states:

> And (We) made your sleep for rest. And (We) made the night as a covering (Q78:9-10).

Tirmidhi transmitted in his *Jami'i* that Khalid bn Walid (RA) said:

> O Messenger of Allah, I cannot sleep at night because of my insomnia. [65] And the Prophet (SAW) replied, 'When you go to your bed to sleep then say, 'O Allah, Lord of the seven heavens and whatever they cover, and Lord of the seven earths and whatever they contain, and Lord of the Shayatin [66] and whomever they mislead, be

---

63. Compare with the Biblical narration, "And Jesus rebuked the unclean spirit, saying to it, deaf and dumb spirit, I command you to come out of him and enter him no more! and the spirit cried out, convulsed him greatly and came out of him" (Mark 1:25-26).
64. *See* detail in chapter six.
65. Insomnia means inability to sleep. It is classified by psychiatrists into early, mid and late insomnia.
66. Plural for Satan or devil.

my protector against all the evils of Your
creation, if any of them oppresses me or
overwhelms me. Whoever is protected by You is
made powerful, and blessed is Your name. There
is no God other than You and there is no Good
except You.

It is also reported that Khalid (RA) complained
to the Prophet of nightmares and the Prophet
(SAW) taught him to pray:

I seek refuge in the face of Allah, the Generous,
and in the perfect words of Allah and I seek
protection from the evil which comes down from
the heaven and displays itself there, and from
the evil which is on the earth, and from the evil
of temptations in the day and in the night and
from everything except whatever brings blessing
with it, O Merciful One.

3.15 Medical and Genetic Counselling

The logical and scientific mind of the Prophet (SAW) enabled
him to confidently inform his companions of the existence of
certain diseases which are inheritable.[67] He also
recommended counselling and proper inquiry on matters
relating to inter or intra family marriages. Evidence of the
knowledge of the familial basis of illness and the science of
heredity of the Prophet (SAW) were reported in a number of
hadith. For example, it is narrated by Abu Hurairah, that:

---

67. It was not until 1866 when an Austrian Monk and Botanist, Gregor
    Mendel (1822-1884) published the results of his research and dis-
    covery of "discrete hereditary elements" (now called genes) that
    the science of heredity was born.

> *One day the Prophet (SAW) passed by and met a father beating his child saying, 'May Allah darken your face and all the faces of those who look like you'. The Prophet (SAW) instantly became annoyed and retorted, saying, 'Surely all faces of mankind bear resemblance to that of their father - Adam. So you should not defame his features.'* [68]

It is also narrated by Abu Hurairah (RA) that:

> *One day a man came to the Messenger of Allah (SAW) and complained that his wife had given birth to a child who did not 160k like him. And the Prophet (SAW) asked him; 'Do you have camels?' The man said, 'Yes'. The Prophet then said, 'What is their nature?' He said; 'They are red camels'. The Prophet then asked him, 'Do you have dark-brown type among them?' And he said, Yes'. The Prophet then asked the man again, Why is that so?' The man said, 'It may be due to ancestral resemblance'. The Prophet then said to him, 'So it is possible that your child has acquired certain features from his forefathers of old'. And the man was satisfied with the Prophet's analogy.* [69]

It was also reported in Sahih Bukhari that the Prophet (SAW) informed one of his companions that it is possible to acquire diseases from parents or grandparents and even

---

68. *See* Fathul Baari Vol.II. pp. 39 and Sahih Muslim Vol. IV pp.2017.
69. See *Bulugul Maram* Vol.II pp 36. Ibn Hajar Al-Asqalani.

domestic animals, such as camels dogs, etc.[70] Therefore, the prohibition of certain consanguineous marriages cannot be unconnected with the scientific mind of the Prophet (SAW) with regards to the knowledge of genetics and the familial basis of certain diseases.[71]

Today, with the recent advances in genetics, there is an increasing awareness of the importance of hereditary factors in the aetielogy and pathogenesis of certain diseases afflicting man. In intra-family marriages, there is every possibility that the couples, if they carry some "abnormal" genes in their body constitution, will transmit them to their offspring. In this way, a particular disease runs through the family tree, causing successive damage and malformation to subsequent generations with all its attendant medical and social consequences. The common diseases that can be transmitted through intra-family marriages include sickle cell disease, diabetes mellitus, asthma, essential hypertension, epilepsy, haemophilia, storage diseases, goitrous cretinism, albinism, Huntington's chorea, myotonic dystrophy, achondroplasia, glaucoma, gout, arthritis, rheumatic heart diseases and certain mental illnesses such as schizophrenia, mental retardation, mania and other forms of psychosis.

3.16   Psychotherapy

Psychotherapy refers to any form of treatment for emotional disturbance or mental disorder for the purpose of removing or modifying symptoms of the disorder, or of promoting character growth and development so as to strengthen the patient's ability to cope with the problems of life. Psychotheraphy includes guidance and counselling,

---

70. This is a pointer to our present day knowledge of Zoonosis, (that is, diseases that are transmissible to man from animals).
71. Marriage between individuals who share blood relation.

behaviour modification, conditioning, psychoanalysis, reassurance and all other forms of treatment in which the major technique employed is communication, rather than drugs or other somatic agents.

Psychotherapy is in reality a form of treatment which directs the patient to recognise his behaviour, to conform with prevailing standards and help in improving the patient to adopt alternative ways of life. Our Creator knows best the make-up of the human psyche and the guidance of the Qur' an and Sunnah is in perfect harmony with human nature.[72] In this field, Muslim scholars and scientists have deduced and developed an extensive and deep knowledge of human behaviour and psychology firmly rooted in the guidance of the Qur'an and Sunnah. In the Qur'an, Allah states:

> *Give glad tidings to those who patiently persevere (over their afflictions), who say, when afflicted with calamity: 'To Allah we belong and to Him is our return' (Q2: 155-156).*

And:

> *He guideth to Himself those who turn to Him in penitence, those who believe and whose hearts find satisfaction in the remembrance of Allah: For without doubt in the remembrance of Allah do hearts find satisfaction (Q13:27-28).*

And:

> *... (it is righteousness) to be firm and patient in pain (or suffering) and adversity, and throughout all periods of panic (Q2:177).*

---

72. Islam is not known for nothing as *Din al-fitrah* (the life transaction of the natural state of man).

Psychologically speaking, every person has two opposing forces at work within him or her. One is the "driving force," which pushes him or her towards some actions, and the other is the "restraining force," which holds him back from others (that is, the *id* and the *ego* instinctive drive). Patience essentially harnesses "the driving force" to push man towards good things, and the "restraining force" to hold him back from actions that are harmful to himself or others. It has been reported in several traditions that Prophet (SAW) employed different forms of what we can term psychotherapy or psychological counselling in treating both physical and mental illnesses. In Sahih Muslim, the Prophet (SAW) was reported as saying:

> *How amazing is the affair of the believer, everything which happens is good for him, when he encounters good times he gives thanks, and that is good for him and if he encounters hardship he is steadfast, and that is good for him.*

Abu Hurairah in Sahib Bukhari also reported the Prophet (SAW) as saying:

> *Whenever a Muslim is afflicted with a hardship, sickness, sadness, wrong, harm or depression - even a thorn's prick, Allah expiates his sins because of it.*

It was reported on the authority of Muqil bn Yasar (RA) that:

> *One day the Prophet (SAW) paid a visit to Fatima (RA) during her illness to enquire about her health and said, 'How are you, my beloved daughter?' She said, 'By Allah! My worries have*

multiplied, my poverty has intensified to an unbearable extent and my sickness has been prolonged'. The Prophet (SAW) then reassured her saying; 'Are you not satisfied that I married you to him who is the first to profess Islam, the most learned and the most forbearing of all?' And she became reassured.[73]

Ibn Abbas (RA) also reported in Sahih Bukhari that:

One day a black woman came to the Prophet (SAW) and said, 'I have (epileptic) sickness and I get exposed, so supplicate to Allah for me'. The Prophet (SAW) said, 'If you wish, be patient and you will be granted Jannat (paradise), or if you wish I will ask Allah to cure you'. She replied, 'I will be patient, but my body gets exposed, so supplicate to Allah that I do not get exposed'. And he did.

It was reported by Ummu Salamah (RA), wife of the Prophet, in a Sahih Bukhari transmission, that Allah's Apostle (SAW) said:

There is no Muslim afflicted with calamity who says, 'To Allah we belong and to Him is our return; O Allah reward me for this calamity and compensate me with what is better for me', but Allah will (answer his prayer and) compensate him with what is better for him.

In another *hadith* from Aisha (RA) through Urwah and az-Zuhri, the Prophet (SAW) said:

---

73. Musnad of Imam Ahmad. Vol. V, pp.26.

No affliction befalls a Muslim but Allah forgives his wrong actions because of it, even if it be no more than a thorn.[74]

Sa'ad Ibn Abi Waqqas (RA) also said:

I asked the Prophet (SAW) who among the people are most severely tried. 'He said, The Prophets, then the right acting people and so on down through various categories of people. Man will be tested according to the strength of his faith. The stronger his faith, the more severe his trials and the weaker his faith, the lighter his trial. The believer will be continually tried until he walks on earth with all his wrong actions forgiven'.[75]

In another *hadith*, Abu Sa'id AI-Khudri (RA) said:

I entered upon the Prophet (SAW) when he was sick and had a high temperature. I put my hand on the cover with which he was covering himself and I could feel the heat of his fever. I said, 'How strong is your fever, O Messenger of Allah?' He (then) said, 'We Prophets are like that; our pain is multiplied, so our rewards will be multiplied'.[76]

Jabir bnAbdullahi (RA) said that the Messenger of Allah (SAW) entered upon a woman and asked her, "Why are you shivering like that?" She said, 'It is because of fever', and cursed the fever. But the Prophet said, 'Do not slander fever,

---

74. Bukhari and Muslim.
75. Bukari transmission.
76. From Ahmad

because it takes away many wrong actions, just as the blacksmith's bellows remove dross and impurities from iron."[77] It was again narrated that Abu Ayyub Al-Ansari (RA) said:

> *The Prophet (SAW) visited a sick man of the Ansar, and when the Prophet asked how he was, he said, 'O Messenger of Allah, I have not closed my eyes for seven days'. The Prophet (SAW) told him, 'Have patience my brother, for if you do, you will be rid of your wrong actions as easily as you acquired them'.*

Anas (RA) narrated that the Prophet (SAW) said:

> *The prayer of the sick person will never be rejected, until he recovers.*

It was narrated by As-Safar in an Ahmad transmission that one day Abubakar (RA) felt ill, so some people visited him and asked whether they should call a doctor for him. He said: 'The Doctor has already seen me'. They asked, 'What did he say?' Abubakar said, 'He said; I do what I want."[78]

Umar Ibn Khattab (RA) was reported saying, "The best days we ever lived were by virtue of patience, and if patience was to take the shape of a man, he would be a noble and generous man." Ali bn Abi Talib (RA) also said, "The relation of patience to *iman* (faith) is like that of the head to the body. If the head is chopped off, the body is useless." Then he raised his voice and said "Certainly the one who has no patience has no *iman*."

---

77. Muslim transmission.
78. He quoted the Qur'anic verse: "Surely your Lord does whatever He wants" (Q11:107), to imply that Allah is his doctor and can make him sick or healthy as He wills.

Thus in Islam, one should not look at sickness only as a gloomy episode characterised with sadness, pains, inactivity and despair, but should also see it as a means of the acquisition of reward, the expiation of sins and a period of repose. Scholars differ as to whether a sick person will be rewarded for the sickness itself, or for being patient during it. However, a majority of the scholars are of the opinion that both the sickness and the patience are rewardable, corresponding to their degrees.

Muslim scholars have defined patience as a positive psychological attitude, by the nature of which we refrain from doing that which is harmful to our lives or the ability of a person to train him or herself to handle difficulties. According to Imam IbnAl-Qayyim in his famous book, *Uddat as-ssabirin wa Dhakhirat as-shakirin (The Equipment of the Patient and the Investment of the Grateful)*, patience has many names according to the situation:

> *If patience consists of restraining sexual instincts and desire, it is called honour, the opposite of which is promiscuity. If it consists of controlling one's stomach, it is called self-control, the opposite of which is greed. If it consists of keeping quiet about that which is not fit to disclose, it is called discretion, the opposite of which is betrayal, lying, slander or libel. If it consists of being content with what is sufficient for one's needs, it is called abstinence, the opposite of which is covetousness. If it consists of controlling one's anger, then it is called forbearance, the opposite of which is impulsiveness and hasty reaction. If it consists of refraining from haste, then it is called gracefulness and steadfastness, the opposite of*

which is to be hotheaded. If it consists of refraining from running away, then it is called courage, the opposite of which is cowardice. If it consists of refraining from taking revenge, then it is called forgiveness. If it consists of refraining from being stingy, then it is called generosity, the opposite of which is miserliness. If it consists of refraining from being lazy and helpless, then it is called dynamism and initiative, the opposite of which is liability or redundancy. If it consists of refraining from blaming and accusing other people, then it is called chivalry or inanliness, the opposite of which is paranoia or delusion.[79]

---

79. Imam Ibn Qayyim in his work Uddat-al-Sabirin, narrated the story of Urwah Ibn Zubarir to demonstrate the virtues of patience and putting trust in God. It was reported that when Urwah Ibn Al-Zubiar came to visit Khalifah Al-Wahid Ibn Abdul Malik, his son Muhammad, who was one of the most handsome of men, mysteriously died and Urwah got gangrene in his leg. Wahid sent doctors to him who suggested that the leg should be amputated, otherwise the gangrene would spread to the rest of his body and kill him. Urwah agreed. When the doctors came to perform the amputation, they asked Urwah whether he would like to drink intoxicants to ease the pain, but (he) said, 'Allah is testing me to see the extent of my patience. How could I go against His commands?' And the doctors began to remove his leg, using a saw. When the saw reach the bone, Urwah fainted and when he came around, sweat was pouring down his face, he was repeatedly reciting *La-ilaha illa Allah, Allahu Akbar!* (There is no deity worthy of being worshipped except Allah, and He is the Greatest).

When the operation was over, he picked up his leg and kissed it, then said, "I swear by the one who mounted me on you, I never used you to walk to any place of wrong action or to any place where Allah would not like me to be." Then he gave instruction that leg should be washed, perfumed, wrapped in a cloth and buried in the Muslim graveyard.

When Urwah left Khalifah Wahid and returned to Medina. His family and friends went to meet him at the outskirts of city and offer their condolence. The only reply he made was to quote from the Qur'an "...truly, we have suffered much fatigue at our journey" (Q18:62) and he did not say more than that.

In the Qur'an, Allah has made patience a condition of receiving many blessings, His protection, love, help and support and standard of courage and determination.

> *And no one will be granted such goodness except those who exercise patience and self-restraint - none but persons of great good fortune (Q41 :35).*

Thus, patience is the central focus of Islamic psychology and the root of Islam itself. It is one of the greatest tool or defense mechanisms in stressful situations that lead to psychological breakdown and psychiatric disorders. Patience is mentioned in the Qur'an about ninety-nine (99) times and is obligatory according to the consensus of scholars.

3.17 Conclusion

In a society where family values are failing apart, divorce, sexual pervasion, substance abuse and addiction are on the increase as ever, and where the idea of the "survival of the fittest," instant satisfaction and the cult of the "superman" prevails, resentment, anxiety, depression, the fear of insecurity and suicide cannot be easily avoided by a series of motivational books or "black and white" tablets. In contrast, Islam channels man into seeking perfection for the sake of Allah and teaches man to seek His help in doing so. This is necessary in order to curb the increasing sense of fear, insecurity, crime, mental illnesses and psychological disorders.

Again in direct contrast to the Western focus on the "self', Islam tells man to look beyond the "self' and focus on Allah. By doing so, man will move towards fulfilling the purposes for which he was created, and therefore attain peace with his Creator, with himself and other created beings. Hence, Islam teaches *tawakkul*[80] (putting one's trust in Allah) and *sabr*

---

80. "Whoever wishes to be the strongest among men, let him put his complete trust in Allah," *hadith*.

(patience, forbearance, fortitude), which enables man to face hardship with dignity and to accept times of ease without becoming arrogant, confused or depressed, thereby providing answers to many psychological problems that trouble mankind today.

In view of the guiding light of the Qur'an, it is worthy to mention a research programme that was recently started at the Akbar Clinic and Institute of Islamic Medicine for Education and Research at Panama City in United States of America. During the research, healthy volunteers were monitored for a variety of physiological and psychological changes or responses while listening to the Qur'anic recitations.

According to the available data "there is a definite and obvious stress reducing effect of the Qur'an on the various organs of the body, possibly through the central and autonomic nervous systems." The physiologic effects of the Qur'an are (from the experiment) achieved through two mechanisms:

i.   Through the meaning of the Qur' an for those who understand the Arabic text.

ii.   Through the sound of the Arabic Qur'anic words for those who do not understand their meaning.

This is only a tip of the iceberg, for Dr Ahmed Elkadi said that:

> *There is good reason to assume that the Qur'an would have a favourable effect on the immune system. This is based on the already known fact that prolonged stress leads to impaired immunity. Conversely, the relief or reduction of stress is expected to improve immunity, and*

*the Qur'an is already known to reduce stress
and its manifestations.*

In view of the findings of this research, verses of *Targheeb* (which promise paradise and other bounties) can be utili sed in *ruqya* for the treatment of mood disorders, such as depression, anxiety, etc. Similarly, verses of *Tarheeb* (verses which foretell about punishment and hell fire) are likely to be effective in treating psychosis, mania, schizophrenia, etc.

Another promising work is that of Dr M. Z. Azhar of the University of Malaysia, who adopted religious psychotherapy (using the Qur' an and Sunnah) in the treatment of anxiety, dysthymic disorders and bereavement with successful results. Another group of researchers from the University of Georgia, in the United States of America also advocates the adoption of Islamic guidelines in stress management in order to· prevent the development of Coronary Artery Disease (CAD).[81]

Therefore, Islamic principles and ideals which are based on Qur' an and Sunnah are the best form of prevention and treatment of psychological

and psychiatric disorders. Hence, it is high time that Muslim physicians and mental health professionals incorporate the Islamic values and ethics in the techniques of psychotherapy.

*It is He (Allah) Who sent down tranquillity into
the hearts of the believers (Q48:4).*

---

81. *See the Journal of Islamic Medical Association of North America.* Vol.32, No.2. April 2000, pp. 57-67.

CHAPTER FOUR

Health Policies

4.1 Family Health and Breast Feeding

According to the Qur'an, one of the most inalienable rights
of the child is the right to life and equal life chances (Q6:151,
17:23,31:14). The spiritual welfare, educational needs and
general well-being of the child must be provided, according
to the Qur'an and Sunnah. Concerning breast feeding, the
Qur'an commands:

> *Mothers shall breast feed their offspring for two*
> *whole years for those who want to complete the*
> *breast feeding. (Q2:233).*

Medically, it is known that human breast milk apart from
its nutritive value, which is vital for the foundational growth
and development of babies, also contains various elements
and antibodies that provide protection against certain diseases
and infections. It is recently established that prolonged breast
feeding encourages both mental and physical development
of children and protects them from diarrhoeal diseases,
respiratory and urinary tract infections, thereby reducing

the rate of morbidity and mortality among neonates, infants and children.

According to a cohort study of 264 children aged 9-18 months in Kenya, in which three groups were defined according to the duration of breast feeding, short, medium and long duration, it was shown that children in the long duration group (on breast feeding) gained more weight and grew faster in comparison to children on short and medium duration breast feeding.

Related studies conducted in Brazil, Gambia, Ghana, Pakistan, Philippines and Senegal on the protective effect of breast feeding in infants and children reveals that "the risk of death from diarrhoea and respiratory infections decreased with age in the first twelve months," and that in contrast, the risk of death in a non-breast-fed infants was found to be higher (about six-fold) than in breast-fed infants. It was also found out that this protective effect of breast milk against diseases and infections persists even in the second year after birth.

It may not be unconnected with the findings of these researches and several other studies in different parts of the world, that the World Health Organisation Collaborative Study Team on the Role of Breast feeding on the Prevention of Infant Mortality now recommends breast feeding to the age of two years! This is a conclusion reached almost at the zenith of man's intellectual and scientific development in the 21st century. Yet, the Prophet (SAW) through divine inspiration has already communicated this simple and sublime information 1400 years ago! Concerning child spacing, it is allowed on health grounds of both the mother and the child:

No soul shall have a burden laid on it greater than it can bear. No mother shall be treated unfairly on account of her child, nor father on account of his child. But fear Allah and know that Allah sees well what you do.[82] *(Q2:233).*

Contraception was also said to be practised during the Prophet's time. Jabir (RA) narrated in the Sahih Bukhari collection that, "We practised *azl (coitus interruptus)*[83] during the time of the Messenger of Allah (SAW). He came to know about it, but he did not prohibit it."

However, birth control (on the basis of population explosion and economy) is discouraged in Islam.[84]

Kill not your children for fear of want We shall provide sustenance for them as well as for you (Q.17:3).[85]

4.2 The Provision of Adequate and Potable Water

Concerning water purification and supply, the Qur'an states:

And We send down from the sky pure water (Q25:48).

This verse specifically signifies the purity of water from pollutants, whether organic or inorganic, one of its essential requirements or characteristics, as distinct from its

---

82. See also Qur'ran 31:14.
83. Means interrupting the process of sexual intercourse by withdrawal of the penis and allowing spillage of the semen outside the vagina.
84. For details see chapter seven.
85. *See* also Qur'an 6:151.

abundance. Concerning its treatment, storage and utility, the Qur'an further states:

> As to the righteous, they shall drink of a cup mixed with **Kafur**; - a fountain where the devotees of Allah do drink, making it flow in unstinted abundance (Q76:5-6).

And:

> They will be given to drink there of a cup mixed with **Zanjabil**, - a fountain there called **Salsabil** (Q7 6: 17).

It is noteworthy that *kafur* (camphor) and *zanjabil* (ginger) are soothing tonics in Eastern medicine, which are added in minute doses to produce an agreeable odour and flavour. This implies that it is permissible or even recommended for man to treat his drinking water with some chemical compounds in order to elevate it to a higher level of excellence in imitation of Allah's Sunnah. The fountain mentioned twice in the preceding two verses implies a spring of water from an underground storage source or one that supplies drinking water in a public place.

Jabir (RA) reported in Sahih Bukhari that, "Once the Prophet (SAW) was thirsty and he said, "If you have any water that has been left standing in a leather or container, I will drink that but if not, then I will drink direct." He also said, "The best drink in this world and in the next is water."

4.3 Legislation on Foods, Drinks, Recreation and Sex

The Qur'an states:

O you people! Eat of what is on earth, lawful and good and do not follow the footsteps of Satan (Q2: 168).

And:

O ye who believe! Eat of the good things that We provided for you, and be grateful to Allah, if it is Him you worship (Q2: 172).

And:

He (Allah) has only forbidden you dead meat, and the blood and the flesh of swine, and that on which any other name has been invoked besides that of Allah. But if one is forced by necessity, without wilful disobedience nor transgressing due limits, then he is guiltless, for Allah is oft-forgiving, Most Merciful (Q2: 173).

Islamic prohibition regarding foods, drinks and sex includes:

* All kinds of intoxicating wines, liquors and hard drugs (Q2:219, 4:43, 5:93).

* Meat and products of swine (pork, ham, lard) and of dead animals and birds that are not properly slaughtered (Qur'an 2: 172-173,5:4).

* All forms of gambling and vain sports (Q2:219, 5:9394).

* All sexual relations out of wedlock, during menses and all manners of talking, walking, looking and dressing

in public that may instigate temptation, arouse lustful desire, stir suspicion or indicate indecency and immodesty (Q23:5-7, 24:30-33, 70:29-31).

Note however that for circumstantial reasons and cases of absolute necessity, there is flexibility for exceptions (Q2: 173,5:4,6:54).

Scientifically, it has been established that carrion (dead meat) is a reservoir for germs and toxins that are harmful to human health when eaten. Logically, spontaneous death of an animal raises the possibility of the presence of a long-standing pathological process that overwhelmed the animal. Eating such decomposed or decayed meat (of dead animal) which usually manifests with changes in colour, texture, taste and smell is contrary to good health and sound habit - hence the Islamic prohibition.

Similarly, ingestion of blood, which is a carrier of nutrients, toxins and poisonous gases is detrimental to health. Till date, there is no known scientific source that suggests the intake of blood for nutritive value. Rather, being a culture media, it provides a thriving environment for the growth and multiplication of pathogenic microbes. Blood taken from live animal (usually done through venopuncture or suction) is also associated with irritation of the gastro intestinal tract that compromised its normal digestive functions, among other medical disorders.

4.4   The Wisdom in the Prohibition of Eating Pigs and Dogs

The prohibition of certain foods and drinks is not by any means an arbitrary action or a dictatorial decree of God. Yet, it is His right, the One Who created human beings, to legalise or prohibit as He deems proper. Because of His mercy, He makes things *haram* (forbidden) and *halal* (allowed) for a reason. Thus, when the Qur' an describes those forbidden things as bad, impure and harmful, it has a vigilant eye on man's morality and wisdom, on his health and wealth, piety and common behaviour - all of which are invaluable assets in the estimation of Islam. The reasons behind this divine intervention are numerous. They are intellectual and medical, spiritual and physical, moral and mental, social and economic in nature. The sole purpose is to show man how to develop himself according to an upright course of life in order to be a healthy unit in the family and community structure and humanity at large.

Findings from veterinary sciences have backed up the Islamic teaching on the prohibition of eating the flesh of swine. In fact, scientific research has pointed out that the pig is among the animals that harbour the highest proportion of zoonotic diseases. It has also been pointed out medically that pork carries the deadly parasitic worm *Trichinella Spiralis*[86] (the trichina worm), which when eaten, colonises the small intestine and produces larvae which invade the body and form cysts in skeletal muscles.[87]

---

86. The infestation is variably called trichinelliasis, trichinellosis, trichiniasis, or trichinous polymyositis, etc.
87. It has three distinct phases, corresponding to the periods in the life cycle of the worm. The intestinal phase occupies the time of growth and maturation of the initial infection and is marked by intestinal disturbance, nausea, pain and diarrhea. The blood-migratory and muscle penetration phase is characterised by fever, sweating, malaise, intense muscle pain and rheumatic aches. Deaths from toxaemia, respiratory distress or other effects are found to occur during this phase. The third phase is the period of worm encystment in the muscles, which is characterised with pain, facial and generalised oedema and other severe clinical manifestations.
Hence, because of the danger of the worm, a special magnifying glass; trichinoscope, has been developed purposely for the inspection of meat suspected of being infected with encysted trichinae.

114   *Medicine in the Qur'an and Sunnah*

Another deadly zoonotic disease from the pig is the influenza viral disease, which in 1918, after the first world war, killed over 3 million people worldwide. The influenza virus was first isolated from pigs and shares almost a similar characteristic with the AIDS virus (Human Immunodeficiency Virus). Up till now there is no drug or vaccine available that can effectively cure or prevent this disease. It was this virus that was at one time found in chickens in Hong Kong that forced the authorities to destroy almost all the chickens in that country.

Taenia Solium is also a parasitic worm (cestode or tapeworm), which is transmissible from pigs to man. When ingested in pork it develops into larvae in the stomach and spreads to other organs including the brain and develops into cysts. It causes a lot of medical disorders including epilepsy, mental derangement, encephalitis, a staggering gait and hydrocephalus.

Other reasons cited as wisdom for the prohibition of pork are found in the statement of several Islamic scholars and researchers. Ibn Taimiyyah, for example, stated concerning the pig, "Pork produces in man the most filthy habits and characteristics, as the pig feeds on a wider range of substances than any other animal, and it is not repulsed by anything." The famous scholar, Dr Yusuf Al-Qaradawi also said concerning the pig, "Since the pig relishes filth and offal, its meat is repugnant to persons of decent taste. Moreover, recent medical research has also shown that eating swine flesh is injurious to health in all climates, especially hot ones."[88]

---

88. See Al-Qaradswi's *The Lawful and the prohibited in Islam*, Translated from Arabic by Kamal El-Helbawy, M. Moinuddin Siddiq'ui, Syed Shukry. Chapter 2 pp.44.

Medically speaking, pork meat is known to contain high levels of cholesterol and lipids, which when eaten lead to development of atherosclerosis. This is risk factor for the development of hypertensive disorders, cerebrovascular accident (stroke), coronary heart disease and sudden death.

Pig is a dirty animal with repulsive habits and characteristics. It is a common sight to see a pig playing in, and even eating, its own excrement. These and many other reasons unmentioned or yet to be discovered constitute just a part of the wisdom in the Islamic prohibition on the consumption of pork.

> *Surely this Qur' an guides to the way that is straightest... (Q17:9).*

Say:

> *The good things are permitted you ... (Q5:4).*

Concerning dogs, there are several scientific researches which shed light on the dangers associated with its consumption as food. It is well known that the dog, like the pig, is a host to many zoonotic diseases among which are ancylostomiasis, leptospirosis, amoebiasis, babesiosis, ascariasis, taeniasis, etc. *Taenia Echinococcus* (adult worm) lives in the dog's intestine and man is infected by the ingestion of the meat containing eggs or dog's excrement. These become embryo in the human small intestine, pass through the blood stream to several organs of the body, including the lung, bones, brain, etc. In 80% of cases the larval stage of the parasite gains access to the liver and develops progressively into a hydatid cyst, which is associated with several complications such as jaundice, calcification, rupture, suppuration, shock, peritonitis and anaphylaxis, etc. It is on account of this that the famous surgeon, Professor Jose Plancoy Fortacin, said:

> *It is the onset of complications (in hydatid cyst) that makes the disease not much inferior (less) to that of a cancerous (malignant) disease.*

Other diseases of dogs transmissible to man include *Diphyllobothrium Mansoni, Multiceps Multiceps, Dipylidium Caninum* and rabies. Rabies is a fatal viral disease caused by rhabdovirus, which is conveyed by the saliva of dogs through bites, licks or abrasions on intact mucous membranes. The disease is associated with fever, cardiac and respiratory failure, paraesthesia, anxiety, excessive salivation, mental depression, weakness, restlessness, hydrophobia, delusions, hallucinations, cranial nerves paralysis and other brain disorders. Death as a result of the respiratory complications of coma, in untreated cases, usually follows about seven (7) days after the onset of symptoms. Furthermore, Al-Qaradawi in his book, *The Lawful and The Prohibited in Islam*, quoted the famous German scientist, Dr Gerard Finstimer, who presented some scientific observations relating to dogs as follows:

> *From the medical point of view the hazards to human health and life from keeping and playing with dogs are not to be ignored. The tapeworm carried by dogs is a cause of chronic disease, sometime resulting in death. Biologically the developmental process of this worm has some unique characteristics. In the lesions caused by them, one worm gives rise to many worms which spread and form other (worms) and varied kind of lesions and abscesses. In human beings the*

size of the abscess may reach that of the head of an infant, while the liver of the infected person or animal may grow 5 to 10 times its normal size. In the infected human it may cause diverse kinds of inflammations in the lungs, muscles, spleen, kidneys and brains and appears in such different forms that specialists, until very recently, had difficulty in recognising it.

The observation went on:

What is worse (about this disease) is that, in spite of our knowledge of its life history, origin and development, we have not been able to devise a cure for it, except that in some rare instances these parasites die out (possibly as a result of the destructive effects of the antibodies, produced in the human body, on them) but not without causing damage. Moreover chemotherapy (drugs) has failed to produce any benefit, and the usual treatment is surgical removal of the abscess.

Finally, Dr Finstimer advised:

For all these reasons we should use all possible resources to fight against this dreadful disease and save man from danger. Man can protect his life and health by keeping a safe distance from dogs. He should not hug them, play with them or let them come close to children. Dogs should not be permitted to lick children's hands or come to places where they play. Dogs must have their

> *own separate bowls and must not be allowed to
> lick bowls and plates used by humans. In
> general, great care must be taken that they do
> not come in contact with anything which is used
> by people for eating and drinking.*

However, little did the medical scientists of the world knew that almost 14 centuries ago the Prophet of Islam (SAW) had forbidden his followers to eat or mix with dogs, and that he warned against their licking plates and against keeping them without necessity. In an authentic narration reported by Abu Hurairah in Sahih Bukhari, the Prophet (SAW) said: The Prophet (SAW) further said:

> *If dogs were not a nation (Ummah) among
> nations, I would have ordered that they be
> killed.*[89]

It should also be noted that the prohibition of keeping dogs in the house does not mean that dogs may be treated cruelly or that they should be eradicated. In fact, the Prophet himself has permitted keeping dogs for genuine purposes (such as hunting, rearing or for guarding). He has also commanded all his followers to be merciful to all animals, including dogs. In one narration reported by Bukhari, the Prophet (SAW) gave a story of a man who assisted a thirsty dog by providing it with water from a well, and the Prophet concluded the story by saying, "Allah appreciated his (service) and forgave the man all his sins."

---

89.   The *hadith* above was said by the Prophet (SAW) following angel Gabriel's remark that angels do not enter a house in which there is a dog. The statement of the prophet (SAW) on recognizing dogs as a nation is in remembrance Qur'an, "There is dogs is not an animal (that lives) on the earth, nor a being that flies on its wings, but (forms part of) communities like you" (Q6:38).

In Islam, the prohibition of keeping dogs without necessity (merely as pets) is also not without reasons, which are based on the health, physical, economic and spiritual well-being of man. Some Muslim scholars are of the opinion that the reason may be because dogs bark at visitors, scare away the needy, chase children (who may fall and get injured) and bite passers-by. On the economic aspect, we observe how lavishly the wealthy people treat their dogs by even including them in their wills. Yet a greater amount of that lavishly spent money can be utilised in the provision for and the improvement of the lives of fellow human beings (neighbours and relatives and the poor), who are dying daily from disease, hunger and poverty.

On the spiritual aspect, scholars said dogs kept for genuine purposes, such as hunting, the guarding of property, cattle or crops, the detection of criminals or chasing thieves away, etc, are not included in the above ruling (Allah knows best). Otherwise, it is not permissible to keep dogs in houses as mere pets with no beneficial service because from the statement of Allah's Messenger (SAW), angels do not enter such houses. In other narrations, the Sunnah has confirmed that evil jinns or devils sometimes take the forms of dogs and cause spiritual havoc. Moreover, we find the Bible addressing certain animals as the abode of evil spirits:

> *So when they (the evil spirits) had come out they went into the herd of swine (Matt. 8:32).*

However, the full understanding of these facts resides within the realm of spiritual knowledge, and science may not (as for now) fully grasp its meaning. Perhaps until when scientists have fully unravelled the mysteries of the unidentified flying objects (UFO), should they be in a better position to appreciate matters relating to spirits.

Finally, we ask the question, how is it possible that the teachings of an unlettered Arab, Muhammad, should agree with the latest findings of scientific research? Surely the answer is in the words of the Qur'an:

Nor does he (Muhammad) say (aught) of (his own desire), it is no less than inspiration sent down to him (Q53:3-4).

Thus, in the light of latest scholarship in the medical and veterinary sciences, we now appreciate the scientific basis behind the prohibition of certain types of food, meat and drink. This harmony between scientific data and divine guidance will further guide those who appreciate truth to submit and surrender wholeheartedly to God's message. This message was perfectly conveyed by his noble Messenger (SAW), whom the Qur'an describes as the "best specimen" for mankind based on his remarkable qualities and value judgement between what is good and what is evil.

He allows them as lawful what is good (and pure) and prohibits them from what is bad (and harmful) (Q7: 157).

It is the appreciation of this wisdom which finds translation in the fields of medical science that makes us bow down in humility and servitude to Him, Who created us and knows best what befits us.

O my Lord! Ordain for us that which is good in this life and in the hereafter for we have turned unto You (Q7: 156).

4.5 Noise as Pollution The Qur'an states:

And be moderate in your pace and lower your voice for the harshest of sound without doubt is the braying of an ass (Q31:19).

The verse above expresses the concept of the "Golden mean"- which is the pivot of the philosophy of Islam - that is, moderation in all things, otherwise your mind and body will be exposed to harm and pollution.

4.6 The Promotion of Medical Ethics

The Qur'an and Sunnah laid down guidelines which govern the practice of medicine and patient's care. These moral values include politeness, patience, humility, cleanliness, compassion, respect, confidentiality, etc. The Qur'an states:

> *... and swell not your cheek (for pride) at men nor walk in insolence through the earth, for Allah loves not any arrogant boaster (Q31:18-19).*

And:

> *And pursue not that of which you have no knowledge; for surely the hearing, the sight and the heart - all of those shall be questioned of (Q17:36).*

In many places also, the Qur'an lay emphasis on the relationship with people, whether colleagues, subordinates or superiors (Qur'an 33:35, 2: 177, 3:16,4:36,5:93,17:37, etc). The Sunnah of the Prophet also abounds with ethical statements or codes, which cut across all the sub-divisions of the various professions in the health sector.

On sound knowledge and self confidence:

Whoever gives medical treatment, but is not recognised as a physician, and who thereby causes death, or anything short of it, will be held responsible for his acts.[90]

On neatness and tidiness:

Cleanliness is part of faith.[91]

On politeness and humility:

The servant of Allah who shows humility, Allah elevates him in the estimation of the people.[92]

On modesty:

Each religion has a virtue of its own, and the virtue of Islam is modesty.[93]

On compassion and tolerance:

The similitude of believers with regard to mutual love, affection and fellow-feeling, is that of one body, when one limb of it aches, the whole body aches.[94]

On confidentiality:

Whoever keeps the secrets of his brother, Allah will cover his secret in this world and the next.[95]

---

90. Transmitted by Abu Dawud, Nasa'i and Ibn Majah.
91. Transmitted by Sahih Muslim.
92. Abu Hurairab reported it.
93. From Sa'id bn Talha.
94. From Nu'man bn Bashir.
95. Cited in Ihya'u Ulumiddin.

Thus, the Islamic code of conduct for Muslims in general and medical or health workers in particular has no comparative.[96]

It epitomises the highest level of morality, that is, the relationship between man and God and between man and other fellow human beings. In Islam, service rendered to other fellow beings will be solely rewarded by Allah, in contrast to the secular concept of personal satisfaction being the reward of the health worker.

4.7 Magic, Witchcraft, Enchantments and Charms

The Qur'an states:

> ... but the devil disbelieved, teaching men magic (Q2: 102). And the magician will never be successful whatever amount (of skill) he may attain (Q20:69).

---

96. Compare with the Physician's oath (also called the Hippocratic Oath) which new doctor takes as mark of their solemnization into the medical profession, which reads:

   "I solemnly pledge to consecrate my life to the service of humanity; I will give to my teacher the respect and gratitude which are their due; I will practice my profession with conscience and dignity; the health of my patient will be my first consideration;

   I will respect the secret which are confided in me. Even after the patient has died. I will maintain by all means in my power, the honor and the noble traditions of the medical profession; My colleagues will be my brother; I will not permit consideration of religion, nationality, race, party politics or social standing to intervene between my duty and my patience; I will maintain the utmost respect for human life from the time of conception; even under threat, I will not use my medical knowledge contrary to the laws of humanity; I make these promise solemnly, freely and upon my honour

In the Sahih Muslim, Abdullahi bn Mas'ud (RA) was reported from what he heard from the Messenger of Allah (SAW) as saying, that, "Anyone who goes to a diviner, a magician or a soothsayer asking something and believing in what he says, denies what was revealed to Muhammad."

Thus, Islam condemns not only the practices of divination, magic and soothsaying but even consulting them for medicinal remedies, healing, harming someone or seeking protection from illness or misfortune. Concerning those who learn these evil practices, the Qur'an states:

> *And they learned (only) what harmed them and what did not benefit them (Q2: 102).*

4.8 Euthanasia (Mercy Killing)

This refers to the painless termination of the life of a person suffering from an incurable disease or intractable pain by medical personnel with or without that person's consent. Euthanasia, popularly known as "mercy killing" or "easy death," involves actions that serve to cause or hasten death, either actively or passively, such as administering an overdose of a drug or withdrawing life support systems from a patient (active or positive euthanasia) or withholding medical treatment that might prolong life, such as the refusal to transfuse a patient who is bleeding (passive or negative euthanasia).

Presently there is a lot of controversy regarding this issue even in the World Health Organisation (WHO). In some countries it is practised, while in others (like Nigeria) it is considered illegal. More than 1400 years ago, the Qur'an and Sunnah passed a health policy that solved this problem once and for all. The Qur'an states:

On that account: We ordained ... that if anyone killed a person... it would be as if he killed the whole of mankind. And if anyone saved a (single) life it would be as if he saved the life of the whole of mankind (Q5:32).

With regards to this, Anas (RA) narrated that the Messenger of Allah (SAW) said:

None of you should wish for death with a view to being relieved from the suffering with which he hath been afflicted. However, if he cannot help so doing, let him say, "O Allah! keep me alive as long as life is better for me and cause me to die when death is better for me."[97]

4.9 Suicide

The Qur'an States:

Do not kill (or destroy) yourselves, for verily Allah hath been merciful to you (Q4:29).

Whatever applies to the sins and offence of murder likewise applies to committing suicide. Whoever takes his life by any means unjustly takes a life which Allah has made sacred. The Prophet (SAW) in two authentic narrations in both Sahih Bukhari and Muslim warned that anyone who commits suicide will be deprived of the mercy of Allah and will not enter paradise.

---

97. Sahih Bukhari transmission.

4.10 Healthcare Delivery and Administration

For effective realisation and equitable distribution of health services as well as other facilities of life, the Qur'an states:

> *Allah doth command you to render back your trust to those whom they are due and to pass judgement upon men with justice: noble is that which Allah exhorts you. Allah is hearing, seeing (Q4:58).*

4.11 The Promotion of Health Services

The Qur'an and Sunnah teaches the promotion of health at the individual and society levels through the acquisition of knowledge. It is worth noting that from the very beginning, there has been a continuous appeal to Muslims by the Qur'an to study and advance the cause of science as a sacred duty. The Qur'an specifically pinpoints to mankind the vital information regarding man, nature and the universe, and how they interact for the benefits of man.

> *... We are never unmindful of (Our) creation (Q.23: 17).*

One of such divine directives or pointers is in the study of life and the mechanism of cure. Allah categorically states:

> *We reveal from the Qur' an that which is healing and a mercy for the believers (Q17:82).*

The noble Prophet Muhammad (SAW), explaining the message of Allah (SWT), was reported by both Abu Hurairah and Jabir (RA) as saying, "Seek medical treatment, for Allah has created no disease except that He created its treatment, apart from old age and death."

In order to promote healthcare delivery or services, Abu Hurairah reported the Messenger of Allah (SAW) saying:

> *Whosoever, dispels from a true believer some grief pertaining to this world, Allah will dispel from him some grief pertaining to the day of resurrection. Whosoever makes things easy for someone who is in difficulties, Allah will make things easy for him both in this life and in the next. Allah is ready to aid any servant so long as the servant is ready to aid his brother.*[98]

4.12 The Rehabilitation of the Sick and the Needy

On rehabilitation, the Qur'an states:

> *And they feed, for the love of Allah, the indigent, the orphan ... (saying), "We feed you for the sake of Allah alone: No reward do we desire from you, nor thanks" (Q76:8-9).*

The Qur'an further states:

> *Those who spend (freely) whether in prosperity or in adversity, who restrain (their) anger and pardon (all) men ...for Allah loves those who do good (Q3: 134).*

Buraydah (RA) related that the Prophet (SAW) said, "A man has three hundred and sixty joints. He must give *sadaqat*

---

98. Sahih Bukhari transmission.

for each one of them."

The Prophet's companions thinking that it was financial *sadaqat* (charity) asked, "Who can afford to do so. Apostle of Allah?" The Prophet (SAW) then said, "Heaping earth upon some phlegm is *sadaqat*, removing an obstruction from a pathway is *sadaqat*.[99] Abu Musa AI-Ash'ari (RA) reported in Sahib Bukhari that the Prophet (SAW) said:

> *Feed the hungry, visit the sick and have the captives set free.*

There are many statements of the Prophet (SAW), which enjoin Muslims to help the blind, the deaf, the weak, advising those who are lost and confused, relieving the distressed, the needy and other healthy practices as forms of *Ibadat* (worship).

4.13 The Promotion of International Health

The Qur'an laid down foundations for the unity of mankind (Q7:189), respect and honour to life and property (Q2: 190) and peace, as the normal course of relations with the exchange of goodwill missions and honest endeavours for the sake of humanity (Q8:61, 42:42). Therefore, the Qur'an encourages co-operation among nations for the promotion of the health status of humanity.

> *O mankind! Verily We created you from a single pair of a male and a female and made you into nations and tribes that you may know each other... (Q49: 13).*

99. That is charity

And:

> *And verily this nation of yours is a single nation. And I am your Lord. (Q23:52).*

And:

> *Mankind was one single nation (Q2: 123).*

The noble Prophet (SAW), who best understood divine messages, said:

> *O Lord! Lord of my life and of everything in the universe! I affirm that all human beings are brothers of one another.*

And he also said:

> *All creatures of God form the family of God, and he is the best loved of God who best loves His creatures.*[100]

In addition, the Sunnah of the Prophet (SAW) has demonstrated that there is no discrimination or barrier on matters of health, helping one another and other things that bring mutual benefit. It was narrated by Anas (RA) that, "A Jewish boy who used to serve the Prophet (SAW) became ill and the Prophet (SAW) went to pay him a visit, prayed for him and invited him to Islam and he accepted."

---

100. Cited in What is Islam by Din M.Rana, Taha publishers, London, Chapter 1, pp.4.

It is also related by Aisha (RA) in an authentic narration, that, "The Prophet (SAW) had many illnesses during which several physicians, both Arab and non-Arab, used to come and sit next to him and treat him." This *hadith* further demonstrates that health services among people recognises no barrier, since it is a matter of utmost necessity.

In Islam, all the men are equal whatever their colour, language, race or nationality may be. It banishes all man-made barriers of distinction or discrimination, gives reality to the idea of all humanity being one family of God, brings the message of life and hope and the promise of a glorious future. Islam wants a united humanity under one banner in order to achieve all these lofty objectives.

CHAPTER FIVE

Research and Development

5.0 Introduction

There is a continuous appeal to mankind by the Qur'an to study natural phenomena and the laws governing the constitution of man and the universe.

> Behold! In the creation of the heavens and the earth and the alternation of night and day, there are indeed signs for men of understanding, who contemplate the wonders of creation in the heavens and the earth (with the saying): "Our Lord not for naught hast Thou created all this! Glory be to thee ..." (Q3: 190-191).

> And Allah sends down rain ... this is a sign ...

> And verily in cattle (too) you will find an instructive sign from what is within their bodies, between excretions and blood, We produce for your drink, milk, pure and agreeable. And from the fruit of the date-palm and the vine you get out strong drink and wholesome food. Behold, in this also is a sign for those who are wise.

And your Lord taught the Bee to build its cells
in hills, on trees ... there issues from within their
bodies a drink ... wherein is a healing for men.
Verily in this is a sign for those who gave
thought (Q16:65-69).

From the above, it is clear that the Qur'an commands
and directs mankind towards the study of science and the
utilisation of its benefit for the growth and development of
societies. In the field of developmental anatomy
(embryology), both the Qur'an and Sunnah had specifically
and accurately described certain facts associated with human
development, much of which were unknown to modern
scientists until the 17th century, when Antony van
Leeuwenhoek invented the microscope. Henceforth, the
microscopic world became visible to the human eye. The
discovery of the various and successive stages of human
development has been difficult throughout the history of
embryology. This is due to the extremely small size of the
embryo, especially in the early weeks of pregnancy, coupled
with the unavailability of the means or facilities to see and
study the embryo in the uterus.

Until the discovery of the microscope, scientists in the
middle ages thought that the human embryo developed from
menstrual blood and that the sperm cell carried a fully created
miniature (tiny) human being which is implanted in the
womb. Therefore, they had no knowledge of the various
stages of human development in the womb.[101] Others
believed that the embryo fully originated or developed from

---

101. Though this concept prevails among all physicians even after the
      discovery of the microscope, Muslim scholars and scientists re-
      jected that idea of the embryo originating from the menstrual
      blood and hold their views according to the Holy Qur'an and
      Sunnah.

man's sperm, and which subsequently become developed inside the uterus. These were the popular and controversial scientific views mainly derived from the teachings of Aristotle (regarded as the founder of the science of embryology) and Galen and even Marcello Malphigi (considered as the – father of modern embryology). The controversy ended only around 1775, when Lazarre Spallanzani showed the necessity of both the ovum (female egg) and sperm (from the male) for the development of a new individual. Yet, twelve centuries earlier, the Qur' an and Sunnah had established most of these facts concerning human development, which anteceded the scientific belief held by scientists over the centuries.[102]

---

102. In this chapter, I have specifically made several references to the book *Human Development as Described in the Qur'an and Sunnah*, which contain research papers presented by Muslim and Non-Muslim scholars and scientists who have analyses the Qur'anic verses and prophetic traditions, which are in harmony with recent scientific findings on human embryology.

The book was published by published by the *Hay'at al-Ijaz al-ilmi* (The Association of the Scientific Signs of the Qur'an and Sunnah) as a proceeding of seminars involving such notable and erudite scholars and scientists comprising professors Keith L. Moore (University of Toronto, Canada), G.C. Goeringer (Georgetown University Medical Central, Washing DC, USA), E. Marshall Johnson (Jefferson Medical college, Philadelphia, Pennsylvania, USA); T.V.N. Persuad, (University of Manitoban, Canada), Joe Leigh Simpson (University of Tennessee, Memphis, USA), Abdul Majeed A.Zindani and Mustafa A. Ahmed (King Abdul Aziz University, Jeddah, Saudi

5.1 The Source of Human Creation

On the question of human creation, the Qur'an states:

Let man think: from what he is created! He is created from a drop emitted (Q86:5-6).[103]

In another verse:

From what substance has He (Allah) treated him (man)? From a drop of mingled sperm He hath created him, and then mouldeth him in due proportions. Then doth He make his pass smooth for him (Q80: 18-20).

O mankind! We created you from a single (pair) of a male and a female (Q49:13).

Again:

That He did create the pairs, - male and female from a sperm drop when lodged in its place (Q53:45-46).

In the traditions of the Prophet (SAW), Abdullahi Ibn Mas'ud (RA) narrated that, "When the Prophet (SAW) was asked by a Jewish person, "O Muhammad, what is man created from?" The Prophet answered, "O Jew, he is created from the fluids of both the man and the woman."[104]

---

103. Translation of the Qu'anic verse and *hadith* in this chapter, except otherwise specified, are adopted from Human Development as Describe in the Qur'an and Sunnah.
104. Musnad Ahmad Vol.p.465.

Muslim scholars and commentators said the word *nutfah*, as appeared in the above verses, refers to minuscule drops of male and female secretions, while *amshaj* refers to the mingling of the two fluids, which in modem science refers to the zygote formed following fertilisation (the union of sperm and egg). Though the appearance of the zygote gives no clue as to its constituent parts, the Qur'an has advanced the scientific fact that it is composed of various components and secretions from both male and female reproductive organs.

It is now known that in the male, the semen, apart from providing nutritive and conductive sero-fluid liquid media for the survival of the spermatic cells, it is also composed of various secretions, which come from several glands (seminal vesicles, prostate, cowper's gland and so on). While in the female, several hormones and secretions play a vital role for the development of the egg *ab initio* from the Graafian follicle stage up to fertilisation. Hence, the Qur' an refers to the resultant embryo as a product of "mingled liquids" from different parts:

Verily, We fashioned man from a small quantity of mingled fluids (Q76:2).

In one *hadith*, the Prophet (SAW) further clarifies:

Not from all the fluid is the offspring created.[105]

This implies that fertilization is performed by only a very small volume of liquid. This concept is not only categorically asserted in the Qur' an, but is also repeatedly expressed:

---

105. *Sahih* Muslim.

God fashioned man from a small quantity of fluid (Sperm) (Q16:4).

The *hadith* of the Prophet (SAW) quoted earlier not only explains the verse mentioned above, but also enlightens further that the creation from both fluids is accomplished through special selection.

This fact is confirmed by modern science, which shows that out of more than a million sperm cells (spermatozoa), only one of them selectively unites with an egg to form an individual (except in a multiple pregnancy where two or more may be involved to produce unidentical twins, triplets, quadruplets, etc, otherwise the same rule applies for identical foetuses). Furthermore, even from the female eggs (ova), only one egg is released out of the many that are contained in the ovary, while several others are lost cyclically through menses. Concerning the process of settlement in the uterus (implantation), the Qur'an states:

> We then place him as a drop of mingled sperm in a place of settlement firmly fixed (Q23: 13).

Zindani et *al* in *Human Development as Described in the Qur'an and Sunnah*, quoting Az-Zabidi said:

> The word *'qarar'* (place of settlement) refers to the relationship of the fetus with the uterus and denotes a place in which water settles or collects (which in modern embryological term is referred to as the amniotic sac containing the amniotic fluid), while *'makeen'* refers to the relationship of the uterus with the body of the mother (that is, firmly fixed) or the fixation

and burying of the mingled sperm (zygote) into the muscular layers of the uterus (implantation).

5.2 Embryonic and Fetal Development

Concerning the developmental stages of the embryo[106] and its protective coverings, the Qur'an states:

> *He (God) makes you in the wombs of your mothers in stages one after another, within three veils of darkness (Q39:6).*

From the above verse, we understand that the fetus, formed from "mingled-fluids," is placed firmly at the appropriate site of the mother's womb within an area of water collection (amniotic fluid) surrounded by three layers: the amniotic membrane, the uterine wall and the abdominal wall. It may also mean the three (3) layers of the uterus: the endometrium, the myometrium and the perimetrium (Allah knows best). All these provide the developing child with a suitable place of settlement for its proper growth. The Qur'an further provides a comprehensive description of human development from the time of the co-mingling of the gamete through and beyond the formation of organs (organogenesis):

---

106. The embryo refers to the early stage of human form (including animal) inside the maternal organism. By convention, the life period of an embryo in man extends from the period of cleavage until the eight (8) week of intra uterine life, when its from has virtually become established. Thereafter, it is called a foetus. Thus, the ending of embryonic life by the 8th week marks the beginning of foetal life of the developing child. The foetus displays the beginning of adult features and is protected in the mother's womb like a king in a castle until birth.

We (God) created man from a quintessence of clay, We then place him as a nutfah (drop) in a place of settlement, firmly fixed, then We made the drop into an alaqah (leech-like structure) and then We changed the alaqah into mudghah (chewed-like substance, somite stage), then We made out of that mudghah, izam (skeleton, bones) then We clothed the bones with lahm (muscles, flesh), then We caused him to grow and come into being and attain the definite (human) form. So blessed be Allah, the Best to create (Q23: 12-14).

The analysis of this verse by Muslim and non-Muslim scholars, embryologists, linguists,· doctors and so on, has revealed that these Qur'anic terms *sulalah, nutfah, alaqah, mudghah, izam* and *lahm* stages have remarkably described the exact stages of development and fulfil the prerequisites of scientific terminology. No wonder, Professor Keith Moore[107] said:

As far as is known from the history of embryology, little was known about the staging and the classification of human embryos until the last one hundred (100) years. The Qur' an was the first source to mention these distinct stages of human development. In fact, the Qur' anic system for classifying human development is amazing since it was recorded in the 7th century AD. Because the staging of human embryo is complex; it is proposed that a new system of classification could be developed, using

---

107. He is internationally recognised as an embryology and the author of many medical texts being taught in medical schools throughout the world.

the terms mentioned in the Qur' an and Sunnah."[108]

In another verse of the Qur'an, Allah states:

Verily We created man from a drop of mingled sperm ... So We gave him (the gifts) of hearing and sight (Q76:2).

And:

Allah has brought you forth from your mother's womb and He has endowed you with hearing and sight, and minds (Q 16:78).

And:

It is He (Allah) who has created you and made for you the faculties of hearing, seeing and understanding (Q67:2.3).[109]

It is important to note that all the verses above indicate that the development of the faculties of hearing precede that of sight or vision (eyes) and that the brain develops last. This is another fact also confirmed by modem embryology. Hence, the serial arrangement with regards to this revelation is not a coincidence, but a design in order to lay emphasis on the wisdom of Allah and His knowledge. Had it been other verses of the Qur' an distort this chronological arrangement of the events of human creation, that is, the evolution of the faculty

---

108. For details see Zindani, A.A. et al (1992): *Human Development as Described in the Qur'an and Sunnah.* Muslim World League Press, Makkah Al-Mukarramah, Saudi Arabia, pp.87-92.
109. Note how the chronology of hearing before sight and then understanding is maintained in all the three verses which are diversely located in the Qur'an and revealed at different and varying times!

of hearing before sight and then the brain in that order, then the relevance for which our attention is drawn would have been confined to the wisdom of creation and not specifically the stages of development. But in these verses, the pointer is both to the wisdom of creation and their chronology. This again demonstrates the inimitable and miraculous character of the holy Qur' an.

With regard to the guidance of the Sunnah on embryology, there are several *hadith* to that effect. Abdullah Ibn Mas'ud narrated that:

> *The Prophet (SAW), the truthful and the trusted, told us, 'In everyone of you, all components of your creation are collected together in your mother's womb by forty (40) days and in that it is an alaqah like that, then in that it is a mudghah like that. Then God sends an angel ordered with four (4) instructions. He is told to record his deeds, his provision (future benefits), whether he will be miserable or happy, and then the spirit is breathed into him (that is, the soul is acquired).*[110]

In another *hadith* narrated by Hudhaifa (RA), the Prophet (SAW) was reported saying:

> *If forty-two nights have passed over the conceptus, God sends an angel to shape it and create its hearing, vision, skin, muscles and bones. Then he (the angel) says, 'O Lord, is it*

110.　The *hadith* was transmitted by all the six (6) *hadith* collectors (*sahsh sittah*). For detail analysis of the *hadith, see* Embryogenesis and Human Development in the First Forty Days in *Human Development as Described in the Qur'an and Sunnah*. pp.77.

male or female? And your Lord decides what He wishes and the angels record it.[111]

The preceding *hadith* indicates the following facts:

- The components of human creation are collected together in the first 40 days.

- The first stages of development, that is, *nutfah, alaqah* and *mudghah* are formed and completed during this period.

- The spirit is acquired during the fetal period.

It is now known, from modern embryology, that all the organs of the body are created during the first 40 days and are all formed in the embryo by the end of the first 40 days (5th-6th week).

5.3 Sex Differentiation and Determination

The Qur'an states:

> *He created what He wills, He bestow male and female according to His will (Q42:49).*

And:

> *And that He did create the two sexes, that is, male and female from nutfah when emitted or planned (Q53:45).*

From the above verse and the *hadith* of the Prophet (SAW) reported from Ibn Mas'ud and Hudhaifah, the sex of any

---

111. Narrated by Sahih Muslim, At-Tabarani, Abu Dawud and Ja'far Al-Firyabi (Fathal Barri Vol 11, p.484).

human being is *ab initio* pre-determined by Allah as part of His *qada wa qadr* (destiny and predestination) and this may be before or during fertilisation (co-mingling of sperm cell from the male and egg from the female). However, in both the Qur'an and Sunnah, this pre-determination is not the only factor of sex differentiation. According to the *hadith*, at a certain period during development God sends an angel to further shape the conceptus into its final form and in doing so, the angel seeks Allah's permission on the final sex of the conceptus in conformity or otherwise with the previously preordained sex of the child. Allah grants the permission according to His will and plan.

In the context of modern embryological knowledge, sex determination is governed by genes, gonads, genitalia and gender (of upbringing), each occurring at different stages of human growth and development. It is known that during fertilisation, the (always) X chromosome from the female ova unites with (either) X or Y chromosome from the male spermatozoa. If the X spermatozoa unites with the X ova, a female child results, on the other hand, if a Y spermatozoa unites with an X ova, a male child results and the genetic sex is determined. Thus, it is the man that determines the genetic sex of the child. This fact is also clearly stated in the Qur'an:

> *And of him (man), He (God) made two sexes,*
> *male and female (Q75:39).*

Thereafter further development continues and the second stage in sex determination is the development of the gonads, comprising the testes in the male and the ovaries in the female. This occurs about the 7th or 8th week of embryonic life. Afterwards, the third stage is determined which is the differentiation of the external genitalia, that is, the development of the vulva and the vagina in the female and the penis in the male, at about the 12th week. Finally, further development with regards to the gender of upbringing is more of an artificial event than natural (yet it plays a significant role in the final determination of the sex of the child).

5.4   The Acquisition of the Soul

Concerning the acquisition of the soul, statements from the Qur'an and Sunnah indicate that the spirit is acquired during foetal development.[112] The Qur' an stated that after the developing child has passed through the *sulala, nutfah, alaqah, mudghah, izama* and *lahma* stages, the spirit is then breathed into it, making it an entirely different creature distinct from its previous physical form. There is a unanimous agreement among Muslim scholars that this is what the divine words of Allah imply in the Qur'anic verse, "And then We brought it into being a new creation" (Q23:l4).

This is another area where inspirational knowledge has put paid to the notion of the supremacy of experimental knowledge. Thus, in spite of the recent advances in science and accumulated knowledge from researches and experiments, medical science is yet to provide a clear, comprehensive and solid understanding of what the soul is. In essence, knowledge of the spirit or soul with regards to the time of its acquisition (which determines the onset of real human life or existence) and the time of its final departure from the physical body (which manifest as death) will resolve the mystery surrounding certain things, of which we know very little, and ignorantly refer to as phenomena. The Qur'an has for long diagnosed and confirmed our malady.

---

112.   According to Imam As-Suyuti in this Tibbi Nabawi," All the peoples of knowledge agreed that no soul is breathed into the developing child until after the fourth month."

They ask you concerning the spirit, Say: "The spirit is of the command of my Lord: It is only a little knowledge that is communicated to you (O men!)" (Q17:85).

It is in the light of this limitation specified by the Qur'an, that we can appreciate the lack of a clear cut concordance on the concept of life and death as a whole and the phenomena of sleep and dreams. Muslim scholars have related the phenomena of sleep, life and death to revolve round the concept of the soul. This understanding is based on Qur'anic statements:

It is Allah who holds the soul (of men) at death; and those that die not (He holds) during their sleep: those on whom He has passed the decree of death, He keeps back (from returning to life), but the rest, He sends (to their bodies), for a term appointed ... Verily in this are signs for those who reflect (Q39:42).

And:

It is He (Allah) who doth hold your souls by night, by day doth he raise you up again; that a term appointed be fulfilled, in the end unto Him will be your return (Q6:60).

According to a *hadith* related by Bukhari, the Prophet (SAW) used to say upon awakening from sleep, "Praise be to Allah Who has raised us up after He held our souls, but unto Him is the resurrection."

Concerning death, there is no difference of opinion among Muslim scholars that once the soul has departed the physical body, it is defined. However, the physical manifestation of the departure of the soul apart, the knowledge of when and how it departs remains obscure and subject to many interpretations. For instance, there is a *hadith* which is said to have advised on the "immediate" disposition of the corpse (following death), yet the 'immediacy' meant by the Prophet (SAW) enjoys no conventional definition among scholars.

In medical science, though the signs of life are well known even to a district health worker, a proper and clear-cut definition of death remains relative and not absolute. Hence, a village health worker can pronounce and certify a person dead only to be confirmed alive in a sophisticated health centre with advanced medical facilities (such as a stethoscope, an electroencephalogram, electrocardiogram, life support machines and so on).[113]

---

113. In the United States, for examples, a presidential commission noted in 1981 that a uniform Determination of Death Act be adopted by all states, an action endorsed by the American Medical Association and American Bar Association. The act reads: "An individual, who has sustained either (1) irreversible cessation of circulatory and respiratory functions; or (2) irreversible cessation of all function of the entire brain, including the brain stem, is dead. A determination of death must be mad in accordance with accepted medical standards."

No wonder then that, as a result of this uncertainty surrounding death, several terms sprang up (such as apparent death, brain death, functional death, somatic death, instantaneous death, etc) all in an attempt to provide a conventional definition for death.

5.5 The Completion of Creation, Labour and Delivery

Concerning the process of labour and delivery, the Qur'an states:

Then He (Allah) made the passage (through the birth canal) easy (Q80:20).

Medical science up till date could not reveal the actual explanation behind the processes that initiate or govern labour, involves the descent of the foetus, its expulsion from the uterus, the rotation or manoeuvres the foetus goes through and the expansion of the pelvic bones among other remarkable events. It is now known that there are various factors (hormonal, uterine contractions, amniotic sac and mechanisms of labour) which synergistically facilitate the passage of the baby by an ordained mechanism best known to God Himself!

5.6 Conclusion

From the above treatise, it is clear that 14 centuries ago the Qur'an and Sunnah collectively gave a detailed and accurate account of human development, knowledge of which was unknown to scientists until the middle of the 17th century. For example, Muslims had from the time of Caliph Vmar (RA) established that a six-month old pregnancy contained a live foetus, but only recently, with advances in prenatal healthcare and embryology, has it been accepted that a 26 week pregnancy (six months) indeed contains a full person. The celebrated embryologist, Professor Keith Moore of the University of Toronto, commenting on the Qur'anic descriptions of embryological development, stated as follows:

The Qur'anic, terms describe accurately the events that occur during the various stages of human development. In fact the Que' anic system for classifying human development is amazing since it was recorded in the 7th century AD.

Another scientist Maurice Bucaille, a French medical doctor, conducted scientific research on Islamic scriptures, expressed the astonishing uniqueness of the Qur'an. He said:

These scientific considerations, which are very specific to the Qur' an, greatly surprised me at first. Up until then I had not thought it possible for one to find so many statements in a text compiled more than thirteen centuries ago referring to extremely diverse subjects and all of them totally in keeping with modem scientific knowledge. In the beginning I had no faith whatsoever in Islam.[114]

Dr Maurice Bucaille, in his search for truth, carried out an extensive and intensive study of the Qur' an from a purely scientific point of view, and confessed in his book, *The Bible, The Qur'an and Modem Science* as follows:

It is inconceivable for a human being living in the 7th century A.D. to have expressed assertions in the Qur'an on highly varied subjects that do

---

114. He, however, accepted Islam and became one of its proponents. This makes true Allah's promise: "Those who strive in our (cause), we will certainly guide them to our paths: for verily Allah is with those who do right" (Q29:69).

not belong to his period and for them to be in
keeping with what was to be revealed about 14
centuries later. For me, there can be no human
explanation to the Qur'an.

However, the truth of the matter is that there is nothing amazing about the uniqueness of the Qur' an because it is the book of Allah, Who is the source of all knowledge.

Our Lord! Thy reach is over all things in mercy
and knowledge (Q 40:7).

And Allah encompasses all and He knows all
things (Q5:54).

Thus, to a Muslim and to any seeker of truth, the treasures of knowledge contained in the Qur' an and the Sunnah of the Prophet (SAW) speak volumes of the divine gift of Allah and the excellent example and legacy left by His noble Messenger (SAW). God Almighty has indeed instructed His Messenger to recognise knowledge as the source of· understanding and wisdom as well as the vehicle of spiritual and material advancement. The Prophet (SAW), inspired by divine power, commanded all his followers to seek for knowledge from the cradle to the grave, and to go even in far away China in its pursuit. In one tradition, the Messenger of Allah (SAW) said:

One hour of studying is better than a night of
praying.

In another *hadith:*

Every disease has a cure. Knowing the right
medicine will cure the disease by God's leave.

This prophetic statement attributing a cure for every disease is a general rule that encourages people to research and understand the medicinal properties needed to cure their illnesses. His saying even goes to the extent of encouraging research of the potency of remedies. Such constant research and trials will also demonstrate physicians' dependence on God Almighty, and expand their horizons in meeting the criteria of the "right medicine" described in the saying of the Messenger of Allah (SAW).

5.7 Reflection

It should however be noted that although the biological or anatomical descriptions and statements of the Qur'an are in accord with the 7 established facts of the medical sciences, the primary intention of the Qur'an is not merely scientific and should not be a subject of scientific scrutiny and assessment. Therefore, the Qur'an is the standard measurement. In other words, the Qur'an can measure scientific information, assess its usefulness or truthfulness or reject its fallacies and errors, and not vice versa (Q15:1, 25:33, 26:2, 27:1, 28:2, etc).

This is because science is based on experiment and investigation, and laws using experiment as their foundation are bound to change and remains unstable. It is also apparent that scientists, whenever they come to an inconclusive finding or "dead end," try to solve the problem by means of various hypotheses, or by postponing its definitive solution until more extensive research has taken place.

For example, until recently, man imagined his being to consist simply of a symmetrical and well-proportioned form; he was unaware of the complex mysteries contained in his creation. Today, he has discovered astounding and far-reaching truths concerning the interior of his being, realising that there are tens of millions of billions of cells in his body. This makes possible a particular appreciation of the greatness of the Creator responsible for this artefact that was not possible in the past. Hence, scientific discoveries and knowledge are not conclusive on matters relating to the universe or man, since they illuminate a limited realm – the knowledge of the part, not of the whole of creation.

The Qur'anic position regarding man, the universe and God are beyond investigative range and scope of scientific methods and instruments. The primary motives of the Qur'an *vis-a-vis* man's creation can be generally stated as follows:

i.   To inform man of the powerful Wisdom and Power behind his creation and design (Q96:1-5, 95:4, 23:17, 12:11, etc).

ii. To inform man of his uniqueness the purpose of his creation and duties (Q30:33, 36:17, etc)

iii. To develop a higher sense of God's consciousness or *taqwa* in human beings. (Q6:2;18:32, 4:1, etc).

iv. To affirm the fact of resurrection, indicating that God who created man *ex-nihilo* (from non existence) certainly can raise him again for the purpose of accountability (Q23:8, 4:2, etc).

CHAPTER SIX

Spiritual Health

6.0 Introduction

Spiritual medicine is one area where Islamic oriented medical science differs from the modern medicine. The word spirit, according to the Oxford Dictionary is the "immaterial part of a person believed to exist forever." It is also defined as "life and consciousness not associated with a body (disembodied soul)." Spiritual health is therefore a dynamic state of well-being that emphasises a proper relationship with the spiritual dimensions of living experience.

Islam recognises and organises the spiritual or moral life of man in such a way as to provide him with all the spiritual nourishment he needs for safety, peace and righteousness. One of the fundamental errors of modern medicine is its mechanistic view of life. This is to say living organisms are regarded as living machines consisting of separate parts. It believes that all aspects of living organisms can be understood by reducing them to their smallest constituents, and by studying the mechanisms through which these operate or interact.

However, it is becoming increasingly apparent that such a mechanistic view of life is not only incorrect, but also inadequate to meet the demands of the health problems of man in relation to his ecological system beyond his ordinary daily life. In other words, this refers to the existence of another world independent of and simultaneous with our world. Although science has taken greater steps forward, there still remains an utter disparity between what man has learned and what he does not know. What is called science and regarded by some scientists as the sum total of reality, is simply a collection of laws applicable to a single dimension of the world. The result of all human effort and experimentation is a body of knowledge concerning a minute bright dot-comparable to the dim light of a candle in a dark night. In short, we know very little of the beginning of our journey, the nature of the worlds and other coexisting species.

Admitting human limitation in research in a world that is vast, Camille Flammarion, the famous scientist, state the following in his book on astronomy:

> *The entire life of humanity, for all the pride man takes in his political and religious history, or even the whole life of our planet with all its splendour, is like the dream of a fleeting moment. If it were desired to write out again all works of research penned by millions of scholars in millions of books, the ink required for the task would not exceed the capacity of a small tanker. But to describe and arrange in orderly fashion the forms of all existent things upon earth and in the heavens, in invisible past ages and in the infinite future – to write down, in short all the*

mysteries of creation – might require more ink
than the oceans contain water. [115]

It is only recently that the World Health Organisation (WHO) admitted this deficiency and made the confession that:

The limitations of a mechanistic view of health
are now becoming apparent and this has been
reinforced by a new awareness of ecology.[116]

However, this honest confession was but a mere repetition of that of Hippocrates, who in prescribing some remedies for epileptic fits, said:

It is useful for convulsions, I do not mean the
type treated by temple priests, but I mean the
convulsions treated by doctors. These
(medicines) are beneficial in the case of fits due
to human and other biological causes, as for fits
resulting from the effects of spirits, these
remedies are of no use.

Hippocrates, also admitting superiority of divine knowledge over experimental knowledge, concluded his statement with the following words:

---

115. This statement is reminiscent of the Qur'anic verse: "And if all the trees on earth were pens and the ocean (were ink), with seven oceans behind it to add to its (supply) yet would not the words of Allah be exhausted (in the writing); for Allah is exalted power, full of wisdom" (Q31:27).
116. See "The Relevance of the Concept of Spiritual Health," In The Medicare medical journal. Vol.5 No.10, pp.11.

Our medicine compared with the medicine of the temple priest is like an old woman's medicine in comparison to our medicine.

We should note that in spite of the rapid advancement of modern medicine through the ages till date, there are some categories of epilepsy which cannot be traced to any known cause, and are termed idiopathic. Thus, the level of man-made scientific inquiry cannot be equated with the knowledge received through divine inspiration. Imam Al-Ghazzali, in *The Confessions of Al-Ghazzali* explains further why religious knowledge cannot be compared with man-made science; He said:

Religious knowledge is based on inspiration which is a degree or level of knowledge above the attainment of scientific certitude, beyond perception of the senses (touch, sight, hearing, etc), beyond reason and beyond experiments. To prove the possibility of inspiration is to prove that it belongs to a category of knowledge which cannot be attained by reason. It is solely derived from the revelations and special grace of God. Some astronomical phenomena only occur once in a thousand years, how then can we know them by experience?

Thus, the extent of scientific knowledge cannot be compared to the divine knowledge or revelations Almighty Allah had revealed to His Messengers (SAW) concerning what benefits man or what may harm him. Of the sum total of true divine knowledge, it is only a small part that ordinary mortals can understand! We are only given that which we can understand, however dimly. So we are not in a position to reject or deny a thing because we are ignorant of it; the absurdity is analogous to a blind man who denies the existence of stars because he cannot see them. This is the same case with some scientists who arrogantly denied all values higher than intellect and reason, and even boast of their ignorant denial. Their claim is based on materialism, which looks at the world with one eye closed and the other opened. Moreover, this notion arises from the failure of some scientists to understand that science illuminates a limited realm, and that the scientific world view is a knowledge of the part, not a knowledge of the whole. The Qur'an states:

> *They ask you concerning the Spirit, Say: 'The Spirit is of the command of my Lord. It is only a little of knowledge that is communicated to you (O men!) (Q17:85).*

Thus, spiritual knowledge is the domain of religions, and science with its inadequate instruments cannot explain matters that are related to spirits. However, that does not mean that the knowledge of spirits is beyond the grasp of science, since experimental science is a developing field and has neither attained its peak or perfection, nor has it claimed to unravel all the mysteries of life; whereas Islam is a divine knowledge made perfect by the Creator Himself. Spiritual knowledge is part of God's manifestation of His existence, and it is right to assume that one day science may uphold the truth of spiritual knowledge as described in the Qur'an and Sunnah.

6.1 The Existence of Jinn, Their Nature and Effect on the Human Body

No one among the Muslims denies the existence of jinn (or "genies" in the West). As for the Jews and Christians, they recognise that jinn exist in the same way that Muslims do. The reason for the widespread belief in the existence of jinn is the continual and consistent mention of their existence in the messages of the Prophets.

The Qur'an states this about Prophet Sulaiman (AS):

And there were Jinn that worked in front of him, by the leave of His Lord (Q34: 12).

About Jesus Christ (AS) the Bible narrates:

And he went throughout all Galilee, preaching in their synagogues and casting out demons. (Mark 1 :29)

The Qur'an also speaks concerning those who worship Jinns:

Yet they make the Jinn equal with Allah, though Allah did create the jinns (Q6: 100).

The jinn were described by the Prophet as independent and intelligent living beings created with free will, dwelling on earth in a world parallel to that of man, invisible to human eyes in their normal state and capable of transformation to other creatures or forms (For example, snakes, dogs, human, etc). The Arabic word jinn comes from the verb *junna*, which means to hide. Consequently, the embryo hidden in the womb (uterus) is *called janeen,* and the heart hidden in the chest *cavity, jaann.* The English word demon for jinn i~ derived from a Greek word *daimon* or *daimons* (plural). In Islam, jinns are not fallen angels, but a special creation of God from the fire of a scorching wind (Qur'an 15:2), whereas the angels were created from light as narrated by Aisha (RA) from the Prophet (SAW). Moreover, unlike the jinn, angels do not have freewill (Q5:6).

However, Satan or *Iblis* who is a jinn (and not a fallen angel) was in the company of angels before his sinful fall and rejection from heaven. Thus, regardless of interpretation of what jinn are, most people in the nations of the earth acknowledged their existence based on countless experience which could not be elaborated here.

6.2 Possession

This refers to the effect of a jinn on a person, particularly when it enters a man and controls him. On whether the jinn have effect on the human body, there is a great deal of evidences. The Qur'an states:

> *Those who devour interest (usury) will not stand except as stands one whom the Satan by his touch hath driven to madness (Q2:275).*

And:

> *True, there were some among men who sought refuge in some among the Jinn but they (the Jinn) only increased their fears (Q72:6).*

The Qur'an further confirms:

> *And if (at any time) an incitement to discord is made to you by the devil seek refuge in Allah.*

He is the one who hears and knows all things (Q41:36).

And about the prayer of Mary's mother, the Qur'an states:

And I commend her and her offspring to Your protection from Satan, the rejected (Q3:36).

And about the Prophet Job, (AS) the Qur'an narrates:

Behold he cried to his Lord: "Satan has afflicted me with distress and suffering" (Q38:42).

AI-Qurtubi, summarising the comments of various Islamic scholars on the first quoted verse (Q2:275) said, "There is proof in this verse that the denial of jinn possession, the claims that insanity has only physical origins and that the jinn does not enter humans nor touch them, are all incorrect. "

The evidence of the effect of the jinn on man is also visible in several Qur'anic verses in which Allah (SWT) refutes and rejects the allegation levelled against His Messenger that he was mad due to the effect of jinn on him (the idea of demoniacal possession is an age-long belief or notion distinctly in the minds of people at the time).The Qur'an states:

Your companion (Muhammad) is not possessed (Q34:46). Thou art not by the grace of thy Lord, mad or possessed (Q68:2).

And (O people)! Your companion is not one possessed (Q81:22).

And:

> *Do they not reflect? Their companion*
> *(Muhammad) is not seized with madness.*[117]
> *(Q7:184).*

In an authentic narration by Anas collected in both Sahih Bukhari and Muslim, the Prophet (SAW) was reported to have said, "Satan flows in the bloodstream of men." Abdullahi the son of Ahmad Ibn Hanbali also said, "I told my father that someone claims that Jinn do not enter the bodies of humans and he said, "O my young son! he lies, for that was one of them (the jinn) speaking with his tongue." The famous scholar Ibn Taimiyyah in his book, *The Essay* on *the Jinn* said:

> *The existence of Jinn and their effects on humans*
> *is confirmed by Allah, the Sunnah of His blessed*
> *Prophet and the consensus of the opinion of*
> *Muslim scholars. Therefore, only ignorant*
> *doctors and pseudo-intellectuals, who consider*
> *heresy a virtue, deny spirit possession and their*
> *effects in the body of the insane. They have no*
> *evidence for their denial except their ignorance*
> *of its occurrence, as there is nothing in the field*
> *of medicine which rejects it, while the senses*
> *and experiences of people worldwide confirm it.*
> *Their ascribing it (that is, madness) to the*
> *preponderance of some humour is correct in some*
> *instances, but not in all.*

---

117. Note that, in all the above verses the original Arabic word jinn is used for demoniacal possession.

The Sheikh went on saying:

Those who deny the Jinn's existence or its effects on the human body, because the beliefs and experimental knowledge of their profession contain nothing which confirms their existence or effects, merely express their lack of knowledge. Such is the case of a medical doctor who looks after the health of the body by treating the physical symptoms of its sickness from the point of view of the changes in its physical make-up without considering what may happen to the body as a result of the effect of the jinn on it.
118

Truly, the soul has a greater effect on the body than mere medicinal remedies. The recognition of this fact in modern medicine has led to the appreciation and advancement of the medical fields of psychiatry, psychology and psychotherapy. Thus, the book of Allah, the Most Greatest and the Glorious, the Swinah of His Messenger (SAW) and the consensus of the Muslim nation acknowledge the possibility of a jinn entering a human and possessing him.

And none can know the forces of thy Lord except He, and this is no other than a reminder to mankind (Q74:31).

---

118. See "Ibn Taimiyyah's Essay on the jinns (The demons)''- An abridged and annotated translation by Abu Ameenah Bilal Phillips, pp. 10-32.

How Jinn Possess Man

Occasional possession of men by the jinn may be due to sensual desires on the part of the jinn, capricious whims or even love, just as it may be among humans. However, possession is most often as a result of the jinn being angry because some wrong has been done to them. Thus, it is to them a punishment for those who wronged them, for example, when humans accidentally harm or hurt them by urinating or throwing certain objects at them or by killing some of them. Though humans may not realise what they have done, the jinn are by nature very ignorant, harsh and volatile with a preponderant disposition towards evil. So they vengefully punish humans much more than they actually deserve. Demon possession sometimes also occurs as a result of horseplay, jest or plain evil on the part of the jinn (such as mischief occurs among humans for similar reasons). The jinn usually dwell in places not occupied by humans, like abandoned buildings, open countries, forests, graveyards, shrines, caves, wells, mines, mountains, islands and places of impurity such as garbage dumps and toilets.[119]

6.3 Exorcism

This is the removal of evil spirits or their effects from humans. Islam has specifically prescribed certain methods of exorcism, and considered other methods illegal and prohibited. In practice, people may be divided into three main groups with regard to their belief in demon possession and exorcism:

---

119. The du'a (prayer) which the prophet (SAW) taught to be said before entering toilet clearly indicates that toilets are common habitats for the jinn. The prayer reads: "O Allah, verily I seek refuge in you from the evil of male and female jinn."

- Those who believe in the existence of jinn, but deny that they can enter man.

- Those who believe they can enter man and remove them by prohibited means.

- Those who confirm the reality of demonic possession and use the permissible methods to exorcise them.

The Basis of Exorcism and Its Methods

Exorcism is one of the permissible healing modalities in Islam because it involves the alleviation of grief and suffering. The Prophet's companion Anas (RA) reported that Allah's Messenger (SAW) said:

> *Help your brother whether he is the oppressor or the oppressed. Anas asked: 'Oh Messenger of Allah! I would help him if he is oppressed, but how can I help him when he is the oppressor?' He replied, 'By preventing him from oppression you are helping him.'*

It is also reported by Jabir and Umar in the *Sahah* collections that when Allah's Messenger (SAW) was asked about certain incantations, he replied, "Whoever among you is able to help his brother should do so."

However, help should be firstly rendered according to the methods prescribed by Allah and His Messenger. For example, Islamically based prayers, words and phrases should only be used in the way they were used by the Prophet and his companions. When commanding the jinn to righteousness and prohibiting it from evil, it should be done in the same way that the human is ordered and forbidden. Whatever is allowable in the case of humans is also allowable in jinn. For example, repelling the jinn might require persuasion, admonition, praise, scolding, threatening and even invoking Allah's curse.

Of recent among Muslim communities (because of widespread cases of demonic possession), a question has been repeatedly raised, "Is exorcism legal in Islam?" It is indeed among the deeds performed by the Prophets and the righteous who have continually repelled demons from mankind, using what has been commanded by Allah and His Messenger. The Prophet Jesus Christ (AS) did it as reported in the holy Bible:

> *And immediately there was in the synagogue a man with an unclean spirit, and he cried out saying, let us alone; what have we to do with thee, thou Jesus of Nazareth? Art thou come to destroy us? I know thee who thou art, the Holy One of God. But Jesus rebuked him, saying 'Be silent and come out of him!' And when the unclean spirit had convulsed him and cried out with a loud voice, he came out of him. And that evening at sundown they brought to him all who were sick and those who were demon possessed. He healed many who were sick and cast out many demons. And he went through-out all Galilee, preaching in their synagogues and casting out demons (Mark 1:23-39).*[120]

In Islamic traditions, there are several narrations regarding exorcism performed by our noble Prophet (SAW) and his companions. Among the many narrated accounts

---

120. Other incidents in which Jesus Christ conduct exorcism were nar-
      rated almost in all the four gospel (for example, Mark 5:13, Luke
      4:35, Matthew 9:32-33, John 9.6).

explaining how exorcism should be conducted, was one collected by Abu Dawud:

> *It is reported from Khaarij bn as-Salt from his uncle that he came to the Prophet (SAW) and embraced Islam. On his return he came upon a tribe which had among them a madman bound in iron chains. The madman's family said, 'We have been in-formed that your companion (i.e. the Prophet) has come with good. Do you have anything to treat illnesses with?' 'I recited over him F atihatul-kitab (the first Chapter of the Qur' an) and he got well. They gave me one hundred sheep so I went back to Allah's Messenger and informed him. He asked me; 'Did you recite anything beside this?' I replied 'No'. He said, 'Take them, for by my religion, whoever eats by a false incantation will fail. Verily you have eaten by an incantation of truth.'*

It is also narrated by Ummu Abaan that her father Alwaazi, said her grandfather, *Az-zaari* bn Amir Al-Abdee, went to Allah's Messenger (SAW) with a son of his who was insane. She reported that her grandfather said:

> *When we reached Allah's Messenger (SAW), I said: 'I have with me a son who is insane whom I have brought for you to pray to Allah for'. He said 'Bring him to me'. So I went to get him and took him by the hand back to the Messenger of Allah (SAW). He said 'Bring him close to me and turn his back to me'. He then grabbed his garment and began to beat him on his back so*

much so that I saw the whiteness of his armpits. While doing so he said, 'Get out enemy of Allah! enemy of Allah get out!' The boy then began to gaze in a healthy manner quite different from his earlier gaze. Allah's Messenger then sat him down directly in front of him, called for some water for him and wiped his face, then he prayed for him. After the Messenger of Allah's prayer, there was none in the delegation better than him.[121]

Ahmad told of another narration from Wakee from Ya'laa bin Murrah that on another occasion, a woman brought a demented son of hers to the Prophet (SAW). The Prophet said: 'Get out of him enemy of Allah, I am the Messenger of Allah'. The boy got well.

In both Sahih Bukhari and Muslim and other *hadith* collections, it has been authentically reported that the Prophet's companions exorcised jinn from people using Qur'anic recitation, and that the Prophet (SAW) also permitted them to take gifts for curing through exorcism.

Imam Ibn Qayyim mentioned that his teacher, Imam Ibn Taymiyyah, told him that on one occasion he read the verse: *"Afa hasibtum Annama Khalaqnaakum Abathan wa annakum ilaynaa laa turja' oon"* (Q23: 115)[122] in a madman's ear and the possessing spirit said in a drained-out voice, "Yeeees". So he (Ibn Taimiyyah) took a stick and beat the man on the veins of his neck until his arm became fatigued from hitting. During the beating it cried out, "I love him." The Sheikh said, "He does not love you." It said, "I want to

---

121. Narrated in Musnad Ahmad and Suhan Abu Dawud.
122. "Did you then think that we had created you in jest and that you would not be brought back to us (for account)" (Q23:115).

make Hajj (Pilgrimage) with him." He replied, "He does not want to make Hajj with you." It said, "I will leave him in your honour." He replied "No, do so in obedience to Allah and His Messenger." It said, "Then I will leave him. "The mad man sat up looked left and right and said, "Why did I come to the honourable Sheikh?" Those present said to him, "What about all the beating you received?" He asked, "For what would the Sheikh beat me when I have not committed a sin?" He was not at all aware that he had been beaten.

Ibn Taimiyyah also used to treat possessed persons with *Ayatul Khursiy* (Q2: 163-4 - the verse of the throne), and he used to order the possessed as well as the exorcist to read it often along with the *Mu'awwadhataan* (that is, the 113th and 114th chapters of the Qur'an).

The Verses Commonly Used in Exorcism

There is a narration attributed to Abu Laila and collected by Ibn Majah in which he was reported to have said:

> *I was sitting with the Prophet (SAW) when a Bedouin came and said, 'I have a brother who is in pain'. The Prophet (SAW) asked, 'What is paining your brother?' He replied, 'He is mentally deranged'. The Prophet (SAW) then said, 'Go and bring him to me'. He went and brought him and sat him down directly in front of the Prophet (SAW). 1 heard the Prophet recite over him **Fatihatul kitab** (the first chapter of the Qur' an), the beginning four verses of **Suratul Baqarah** (the second chapter of the*

Qur' an) and two from its middle.[123] *Then he recited* **Ayatul Khursiy** *(the verse of the throne).*[124] *And he recited three verses from the end of the chapter (that is,* **Baqarah**), *one verse from Suratul AU Imrana (the 3rd chapter of the Qur' an)*[125] *Then he recited a verse from* **Suratul AI-A 'raaf** *(the 7th chapter)*[126] *and one verse from* **Suratul Mu'minoon** *(the 23rd chapter).*[127] *Then (he recited again) a verse from*

---

123. "And your God is One, there is no god but He, most Gracious, most merciful. Behold! In the creation of the heavens and the earth, in the alternation of the night and the day, in the sailing of the ship through the ocean for the profit of mankind; in the rain which God sands down from the skier, and the life which he give therewith to an earth that is dead, in the beasts of all kinds that setters through the earth; in the change of the winds and the clouds which they trail like their slaves between the sky and earth;(here) indeed are signs for a peoples that are wise (Q2:163-4).
124. Allah! There is no God but He, the living, the Self-subsisting supporter of all, no slumber can seize Him nor sleep. His are all things in the heaven and earth. Who is there that can intercede in His presence except as He permitted? He knoweth what (appeareth to His steward creatures) before or after or behind them. Nor shall they encompass ought of His knowledge except as He width. His throne doth extend Over the heavens and the earth and He feeleth no fatigue in guarding and preserving them. For He is the most High, the Supreme (in glory)" (Q 2:255).
125. "Allah bears witness that there is no God but He and (so do) His angle and those endued with knowledge, firm in justice. There is no God but He, The Exalted in power, the wise" (Q7:18).
126. "Verily your is Allah who created the heaven and the earth in six days and then established Himself on the throne. He veils the day with night, each seeking the other in rapid succession: And the sun, the moon and the stars, (all) are subservient by His command. Verily, His are the creation and the command, blessed is Allah, Lord of the worlds" (Q7:117)
127. "Whoever calls on another god besides Allah no evidence for it and his account is with his lord. Verily the disbelievers will not succeed" (Q23:117).

Suratul linn (2nd chapter).[128] *Then He recited further again, the first 10 verses of* **Suratul Saffat** *(the 37th chapter), three (3) verses from the end of Suratul Hashr (59:22-24),* **Suratullkhlas** *(112th) and the* **Mu'awwadhataan (Suratul Falaq** *113th and Naas 114th). After all the recitations the Bedouin got up completely cured without any complaint.*

From the foregoing, the legality and methods of application of exorcism has been demonstrated. With regards to exorcism involving seeking help against jinn by using written or spoken words and phrases whose meanings are unknown - such methods are illegal. If the preparation (amulets, talisman etc.) or chants or recitations contain *shirk*, their usage automatically becomes *haram* (forbidden). There are sufficient cures in what has been prescribed by Allah and His Prophet (SAW) to remove the need for methods involving *shirk* and those who practise it. Though there are varying opinions on the permissibility of using medicine containing forbidden substances like pork and alcohol, there is no difference of opinion among Islamic scholars with acts of *shirk* (ascribing partnership to Allah) and *kufr* (disbelief) because they are prohibited under all circumstances. There are two reasons to note:

- First is that, it may not have any effect, for most of those who treat illness with prohibited means have no success, instead it may worsen their afflictions.

- Secondly, there are sufficient authentic methods of cure as to make false methods superfluous.

---

128. "And exalted is the majesty of your lord, He has taken neither a wife nor a son" (Q72:3)

Therefore, the importance of upholding strictly the practice of the Prophet (SAW) must be emphasised as the Prophet himself said, "I leave two things with you after which you will never go astray: AI-Qur' an and my Sunnah, the two will never separate (from each other) till they meet me at the pond in paradise." Aisha (RA) also reported the Prophet (SAW) as saying:

> *Whoever innovates in this affair of ours (that is, Islam) something not belonging to it will not have it accepted.*[129]

In another *hadith*, the statement continues:

> *For every innovation is misguidance and every form of misguidance leads to the hell fire.*[130]

Furthermore, on the issue of demonic possession and exorcism, late Sheikh Abdul-Aziz Ibn Baaz's *fatwa* (scholarly opinion and judgement), agrees with the previous presentation. The Sheikh narrated a personal experience in which he exorcised a jinn from a possessed Muslim lady in the company of other scholars and her relatives. The jinn who claimed to be a Buddhist from India professed Islam after the Sheikh had preached to it, and left the woman. After which the woman spoke with her own feminine voice in contrast to the jinn's voice, which was a man's voice (that is, masculine).[131]

---

129. Sahih Bukhari transmission.
130. Tirmidhi and Abu Dawud.
131. The details of that encounter was published in the Al-Mujtama of 18th August 1978 as a respond by Sheikh Baan to a public denial of possession and exorcism made by one Sheikh Ali At- Tantawi in his weekly television programme on channel one of the Saudi Television.

The Sheikh in buttressing further the rights of exorcism said it is not a contradiction of Prophet Sulaiman's prayer requesting Allah to give him dominion (over the wind, animals, jinn, etc) not allowed to anyone, and was granted.[132] The erudite scholar, Abu Ameenah Bilal Philips, in his annotated translation of Ibn Taimiyyah's treatise on jinn, said:

> *Suppose that these incidents were not narrated from the Prophet (SAW) and the Prophets before him, or his companions, or the early scholars due to the inability of the devils to possess people in their time, but they did among us. Allah and His Messenger have still enjoined aiding the oppressed, relieving the distressed and benefiting humanity, all of which include exorcism.*

In another *hadith,* the Prophet (SAW) was reported to have said, "The best among you is he who the community benefit most from his service." In both Sahib Bukhari and Muslim there is a narration in which the Prophet's companion AI-Bara Thn Azib reported that, "The Prophet (SAW) commanded us to do seven things (among which is) helping the oppressed." In exorcism there is also the alleviation of grief and the suffering of the oppressed. Allah's Messenger (SAW) is also reported by Abu Hurairah in Sahib Muslim saying; "Whoever relieves a believer of one of the tragedies of this life, Allah will relieve him of one of the calamities of the Day of Resurrection."

Thus, the fundamental principle on the basis of which exorcism should be understood is that it may be permissible, recommended or even compulsory to defend or aid one who is possessed, because helping the oppressed is a duty according to one's ability. We therefore conclude with the Prophetic

---

132. O my lord! Forgive me and give me a dominion not allowed   any-
      one   after me (Q38:35).

words: "Whoever among you is able to help his brother should do so.[133]

6.4 Healing through Miracles

It is narrated by Sahil bn Sa'd in the *Sahah* collections that when Ali bn Abi Talib (RA) was chronically ill and bedridden and also had ophthalmia, the Prophet (SAW) prayed for him and spat into his eyes. He instantly regained his health and his sight became perfect as ever. It was also reported that during the battle of Uhud, a companion of the Prophet, Qatada bn AI-Numan got a blow on his face which made one of his eyes came out of its socket. The Prophet restored it to its place with his own hand, and it was so completely healed that its sight or vision became better than that of the other eye.[134]

It is also reported in both Sahib Bukhari and Muslim that the Prophet (SAW) received a prophylactic warning from a roasted sheep's leg when placed before him, saying, "O Messenger of Allah, do not eat me, I am poisoned."[135] There are indeed many narrations on the miraculous healing by Allah's Messenger (SAW) and his companions, but this does not acquire a prominent feature of medicine in both the Qur'an and Sunnah. The Islamic concept of medicine appeals to reason, knowledge and practice, rather than amulets, charms or miracles. The Qur'an states:

> *And We refrain from sending the signs, only because the men of former generations treated them as false (Q 17:59).*

133. From Jabri and umar (RA) in the Sahih collections.
134. Ibn His vol.II, pp. 82.
135. Cited in Halal wal Haram Fill-Islam-prophet Moses (AS)

In both *sahah* collections, the Prophet (SAW) was reported saying, "There has never been a Prophet amongst the Prophets who was not bestowed with a sign amongst the signs, which were bestowed on the earlier Prophets. Human beings become believers through them, and truly what I have been bestowed was a revelation (the Qur'an), which Allah has revealed to me. I hope I will have the highest number of followers on the Day of Resurrection." Indeed, every Prophet has special miracles to draw attention to his teachings, even though past generations treated signs and portents with contempt, mockery or rebellion.

For instance, one Prophet raised a mountain above his people's head to provide a shade for them, divided the sea so that people could walk along a dry passage between its two halves, cast his stick and it changed into a serpent (a transformation from the vegetable or plant kingdom to the animal kingdom).[136] While a Prophet placed in the belly of a fish for a considerable number of days survived (on dissolved oxygen?) in spite of the degeneration of his evolutionary adaptive structures or mechanisms to aquatic life (habitat).[137] Another Prophet was sent a wondrous she-camel which fed people with nutritious milk for their physical and spiritual growth.[138] A Prophet healed the blind and the leprous and brought the dead to life after cell disintegration or body decomposition had taken place.[139]

Yet, in spite of the many miracles performed by the Prophets (PBUT), they were treated with contempt, mockery and unbelief. Prophet Jesus (AS), for example, in spite of the miracles he performed mainly on cure and healing, was reported to have lamentably confessed the unbelief of his

---

136. Moses (AS).
137. Jonah (AS).
138. Salih (AS).
139. Jesus (AS)

people.

O faithless and perverse generation, how long shall I be with you? (Matt 17: 17).[140]

You who kill the Prophets and stone those sent to you (Matt 23:37).[141]

For John (the Baptist) came neither eating nor drinking, and they say, "He has a demon" (Matt 11:18).

And when the Son of Man[142] cast out demons, they said: "He is possessed by Beelzebub! It is by the Prince of demons that he drives out demons" (Mark 3 :22).[143]

The Qur'an further confirms:

When thou (Jesus) didst show them the clear signs and the unbelievers among them said: "This is nothing but evident magic" (Q5:110).

Before Jesus (AS), a similar treatment and rejection was meted out to Moses (AS):

And Pharaoh said: 'Surely this (Moses) must be your leader who has taught you magic' (Q20:71).

And Moses said to his people: 'O my people! Why do you vex and insult me, though you know I

---

140. Translation adopted from King James Version, Thomas Nelson Inc, Nashville, New York.
141. Translation adopted from the New International Version, Kingsway publications, USA.
142. That is, Jesus Christ.
143. Translation adopted The New International Version, Kingsway publications, USA.

am the Messenger of Allah sent to you?'
(Q61:5).

On the other hand, miracles by themselves are not the objectives of Prophethood, that is, they are not the essential proofs in the final assessment of truth. The Bible reported Jesus as saying:

> *Many will say to Me on that day, 'Lord, Lord, have we not prophesied in Your name? And in Your name cast out demons and in Your name performed many miracles?' And then I will declare to them, 'I never knew you, depart from me, you who practise lawlessness. (Matt. 7:22).*

In another place he further emphasises his point on the meaninglessness of miracles:

> *See to it that no one misleads you ... For false Christ and false Prophets will rise and show great signs and wonders to deceive, if possible, even the very elect (Matt 24: 4 and 24).*

Concerning the healing prowess of Jesus Christ (AS), Allah states in the holy Qur'an:

> *And you healed those born blind and lepers by My permission and behold! you bring forth the dead by My permission (Q5:110).*

It is noted from the above verse how the words "by My permission" are repeated with the mention of each miracle so as to emphasise the fact that they arose not out of the power or will of Jesus, but by Allah's power and will which He performed through him. The above verse is also a fact to which the Bible attests to, for Jesus was reported in many places in the Bible to refer the power and the will of miracles to Allah; the Supreme being over all mortals. (Acts 2:22, John 5:30, Luke 11:40, Luke 11 :20, etc). In many places, Jesus also admittedly told his disciples that the success of miraculous healing depends on the strength of faith and persistent prayers to God. For example, when he was asked by his disciples how it were possible for him to cast out demons, he said:

> *This kind can come out by nothing but prayer and fasting (Mark 9:29).*

The verse above and related statements quoted earlier are in agreement with the Qur' anic stand on miracles. The noble Prophet (SAW) was instructed to respond to the charge of his critics on their demand for miracles as follows:

> *Yet they say: "Why are not signs sent down to him from his Lord?" Say: "The signs are indeed with Allah and 1 am only a clear Warner" (Q29:50).*

The Qur'an further commands the Prophet (SAW) to acknowledge the absolute power of God and His complete and total Lordship over all things, and at the same time confess his own limitations and duty.

> *Say (O Muhammad): "I have no power over any good or harm to myself except as Allah willed. I am but a warner and a bringer of glad tidings to those who have faith" (Q7: 188).*[144]

---

144. In comparisons Jesus said to his peoples, the Jews, "I can of mine self do nothing" (John 5:30).

Therefore, it is understood that healing or cure can be achieved through a miraculous performance, which is a further demonstration of God's power to man through his Prophets and few of His chosen servants. This must also be distinguished from fake miracles performed by pseudo-priests or scholars who are aided by the devil and his evil forces and their spiritual masters. Imam Ibn Taimiyyah in his book, *Al-Furqaan Bay na Awliya' ar Rahman Wa Awliyah ash Shaitaan (Distinction between the Friends of Allah and the Friends of the Devil)* mentioned that:

> *There are many cases of men seeking help from such evil people even with successful results but that does not confer on the performer any authenticity or truth. There are indeed many among idol worshippers, few Christians and heretical Muslims who are driven astray by satanic deception through so-called acts of wonders or miracles. Satan is able to make such misdeeds appealing to them by convincing them that they are among the* **Karamaat** *(supernatural or quasi-miraculous feats of the righteous).*

Imam Ghazzali also clarifies further that miracles by themselves do not constitute a basis for certitude, he said:

> *If for example, anyone possessing the power of changing a stone into gold or a stick into serpent and suppose the man should come to me, when I am firmly convinced that ten is more than three and say 'No, on the contrary, three is more than ten and to prove it I change this rod into a serpent'. And supposing that he actually did so*

(that is, converted the rod into a serpent), I should remain nonetheless convinced of the falsity of his assertion and although his miracle might arouse my astonishment, it would not instil any doubt in my belief or shake the basis of my certitude.[145]

Thus, we conclude that healing by miracles is another facet of remedy and phenomenon which is above the level of scientific certitude and reason, and therefore it strictly belongs to the domain of Prophethood.

6.5   The Use of Washed Qur'anic Verses on Slates as a Medicinal Remedy

It is reported by Abdullahi Ibn Ahmad, who quoted a narration from his father collected from Abdullahi Ibn Abbas in which he was reported saying that, "If a woman has a difficult time in giving birth, write these verses on a slate for her, 'In the name of Allah, there is no god but He the Gentle, the Generous. Glory be to Allah, Lord of the mighty throne. All praise is due to Allah, Lord of the worlds,' and (also write for her) the 46th verse of *Suratul Nazi'at* and the 35th verse of *Suratul Ahqaaf*, wash the slate and let her drink."

In another narration with the same chain of narrators, Ibn Ahmad stated that, "My father reported that Ibn Abbas also said, 'Write it in a clean vessel and drink it'. In yet another narration, he was reported to have added, 'Give it to her to

---

145.   See the confessions of Al-Ghazzali by Claud field, Ashraf publications, Lahore, pp. 16-22.

drink and to sprinkle on her body below the navel.' Abdullahi also reported that his father Imam Ahmad practised it.[146]

Thus, from the above it is permissible to write something from the Qur' an on a wooden slate with an ink made from allowable substances. The writing may be washed and drunk by the afflicted or sick, as has been stated by Imam Ahmad and others, mainly based on the above narration. On the other hand, some Muslim scholars argued on the authenticity of the above *hadith* in favour of other *ahadith*, which came directly from the Prophet (SAW) discouraging the practice. The Prophet himself never performed such practices, as well as his closest companions.

While the Qur'an repeatedly pronounced itself as 'a healing and mercy,' its appeal is more of spiritual and natural than mere ingestion of its material writing or pages! There is preponderence of opinion among Muslim scholars that the use of washed Qur'anic verses off slates for medicinal purpose confers, if any, a psychological satisfactory effect rather than actual remedy. This is because it is not meant for that purpose. However, one cannot disregard the placebo effect of some practices or drugs even if they are unrelated to the malady for which they are meant to effect cure.

Consequently, it seems safer (healthwise in terms of avoiding the unhygienic or unsanitary conditions associated with the practice in the traditional setting and for spiritual safeguard of one's faith) to discourage the practice. Instead emphasis should be laid on research and utilisation of the natural remedies specifically pointed out by the Qur' an and genuine prophetic practice. Allah knows best.

---

146. Other Muslim scholars like AL-Qadi Iyyaad have supported the practice of writing Qur'anic verse on slate, wash and drink it by making an analogy with Nafath (blowing) during incantation and recitation of the chapters or prayers of refuge (that is, al-mu'awwadhatani) which is authentically confirmed by the prophet's (SAW) practice.

However, there is unanimous agreement among the scholars on *nafath* - which is blowing air on the underspread palms during incantation and the recitation of certain prayers or Qur'anic verses. The scholar AI-Qadi Iyyad has suggested that the benefit of blowing air is derived from the blessing in the moisture or air, which has been touched by divine words. Though the benefit of blowing air can only be defined by the one who prescribed it, the Prophet (SAW) himself did not elaborate on its purpose. [147]

6.6   The Use of Amulets and Charms

On the issue of using amulets and talismans, Imam As-Suyuti in his *Tibbi Nabawi* reported that Abdullahi bn Umar (RA) used to teach his children a special prayer for insomnia while they were still young and growing up. He would write down as a text and hang it round their necks. Abu Dawud and Tirmidhi have transmitted this *hadith.* He also quoted Ahmad saying that Aisha (RA), wife of the Prophet, did not oppose the practice. AI-Marwazi reported a *hadith* in which Abu Mansur Amr bn Majma said Yunusa bn Hiben narrated that, he questioned Aba Jafar Muhammad bn Ali about wearing an amulet and he answered:

> *If the amulet contains a divine text or some Prophetic words, do wear it and use it as a remedy as much as possible.*[147]

On the other hand, some scholars cited other *ahadith* as evidence against the use of amulets or charms as a medicinal remedy. It was reported from the authority of Uqbah Ibn Amir that he came to the Prophet in a group of ten persons,

---

147.   See *Fathul Baari* Vol. 10, pp. 161 and Sahih Buhari Vol. 8, p233 no.331 and vol.6, p.495, No.536.

and the Prophet (SAW) accepted the oath of allegiance *(bay' ah)* from nine of them withholding himself from the tenth. "What about him?" they asked. The Prophet (SAW) replied, "There is an amulet on his arm." The man tore off the amulet and the Prophet accepted his oath.[148] In another *hadith* reported from the authority of Abdullahi bnAkin (RA) in Jami'a Tirimidhi, the Prophet (SAW) was also reported as saying, "Whoever wears a charm will be left to rely on it." Isah Ibn Hamza also narrated that, "I visited Abdullahi Ibn Hakim who had a fever, I said, 'Why do you not wear a charm?' He replied, 'I seek refuge in Allah from that."

These teachings of the Prophet (SAW) penetrated the minds of his companions, and they rejected such practices, neither accepting nor believing in them.

However, there is a consensual agreement among scholars that, if the preparation contains *shirk*, their usage is automatically prohibited as there is no difference of opinion among scholars with regard to the prohibition of treating sickness with acts of *shirk* (associating partnership to Allah) and *Kufr* (disbelief), that is forbidden under any circumstance. If the constituents of the amulet or talisman do not contain *shirk*, or Qur'anic verse written in impurities like blood or written backwards, nor a portion of the verse omitted or other things which please satan and the person does not take them (amulet or talisman) seriously or ascribe to them the solution to his afflictions, then according to the opinion of some scholars, they may be permissible.[149] These are not without implications on the faith of both the giver and the user. But for fear of the possibility of *shirk* being involved, even if it is not meant to be so initially, some scholars have discouraged people using such means of treatment even

---

148. Cited by Qayyim in his Tibbi Nabawi. Part III, pp. 329-323.
149. Report by Ahmad and Al-Hakim and cited by Yusuf Qaradawi in his The lawful and the prohibited in Islam." Chapter IV, pp.244.

when considered permissible.

> *We have made alluring to each people its own doings (Q6: 108).*

Therefore, as far as the prevention and treatment of diseases are concerned, Islam has prescribed measures which are well known. The Prophet (SAW) was reported as saying:

> *There is remedy in three (3) things: a drink of honey, operation by a cupper and cauterisation.*

In the present time, these three (3) types of cures include, by analogy and extension, all medicine which are taken by mouth or other routes, blood transfusion, surgical intervention and therapies using radiation heat or electricity.[150]

6.7 Omens and Superstitions

An omen refers to something happening as a sign of good or evil fortune. Usually, it is believed to be a warning signal for an impending calamity or disaster. It is likened to a kind of aura or the premonitory sign of an approaching danger. In spite of our claim to civilisation, drawing evil omens from certain places, times, individuals and the like was, and still is, a current superstition among many peoples and communities. Islam has condemned in clear terms the auguring of omens. The Qur' an states:

> *Your auguring of evil omen is with yourselves (Q36: 19).*

---

150. Imam Al-suyuti in his Tabb Nab'awi, consider the justification of using amulets and charms based on the degree to which trust is placed in their intrinsic power to do good or harm, and the degree to which the wordings conform to Islamic principles.

The Prophet (SAW) also said:

He is not of us who seeks evil omens or for whom evil omens are sought.

It has been related by Thn Abbas that the Prophet (SAW) said:

There will be seventy-thousand (70,000) of my followers – not counting those who refuse to consult soothsayers, who will enter the garden (AI-Janat) because they do not believe in bad omens, nor use cautery, but they rely on their Lord.

Augury has no basis in science or in reality, but a manifestation of the weakness of the mind for being a mere superstition. It is indeed ridiculous and preposterous for a sane human being to believe that a certain person or place, the cry of a bird, the flick of an eyelid can bode something evil. We meet many cases in practice whereby patients ascribe a genuine medical problem (such as epilepsy, stroke, blindness, deafness, etc) to an evil omen, and instead of seeking for a cure resort to traditional healers and spiritualists.

Although many people are affected by this weakness at one time or another, this weakness is removed from the mind of the person who turns to Allah, trusting in Him and not letting such ideas obsess him. In this way, it will remain a mere thought which crosses the mind without affecting his actual behaviour. Allah *Subhanahu Wa Ta' alah* will forgive such.

6.8 Magic and Soothsaying

Islam has condemned and rejected soothsaying, magic and divination and all those who go to the practitioners or ask their help and believe in their superstitions and errors. The Prophet (SAW) was reported in Sahih Bukhari as saying:

> *Whosoever goes to a soothsayer and believes in what he says has denied what was revealed to Muhammad.*

The Qur'an also states:

> *... Satan disbelieved; teaching men magic ... and they learned what harmed them, not what profited them and the buyers of the magic would have no share in the happiness of the Hereafter (Q2: 102).*

Concerning the evil effect of magic on a person, the Qur'an rejects their claims to such power:

> *But they (magicians) could not thus harm anyone except by Allah's permission (Q2: 102).* [150]

Although, the secret arts and evil machinations of magicians and witches may cause psychological terror, Muslims are encouraged to cast off fear and do their duty while seeking refuge in divine power and mercy. Therefore, a true Muslim is not expected whenever afflicted by a calamity or sickness, to start wailing or cursing imaginary enemies, or to consult magicians for cure or protection, instead of seeking appropriate medication from authentic healers.

---

151.   Bukhari and Muslim have transmitted this hadith.

CHAPTER SEVEN

Public Health Issues

7.0 Introduction

It becomes necessary if not essential to address certain special issues and problems which though discussed by scholars at various places and times, remain significantly important not only to medical personnel, but also to the man on the street. This is because these issues live with us everyday, and make a very deep impact upon our lives. "The greater need of our time," according to Justice Cardoza of the United States of America, "is a philosophy that will mediate between conflicting claims of stability and progress and supply a principle of growth". Islam provides both. It bestows upon mankind an ideology that satisfies the demands of both stability and change. Deeper reflection reveals that life is neither rigid beyond change, nor is it merely a process of change, pure and simple. The basic problems of life remain the same in all ages and countries, but the ways and means of solving them and the techniques of handling them have undergone various changes through the passage of time.

The Qur'an and Sunnah embody the eternal principles of a guidance given by the Lord of the Universe. This guidance comes from God who is free from limitations of space and time, and as such the principles governing specific individuals and humanity are eternal. But God in His infinite

185

mercy and wisdom has given us the general principles only, and has endowed man with the freedom and intellect to apply them in every age in the way suited to the spirit and condition of that age. It is through *ijtihad* that the men of every age endeavour to apply divine guidance to the problems of their time. Thus, the basic guidance is eternal and permanent, while there is dynamism in the means of applying it to the particular needs of every successive age. That is why Islam remains forever fresh and modern.

> *For He (Allah) fully knows all creation (Q36:79).*

And:

> *Should He not know - He that created? And He is the Subtle, the Aware. It is He Who has made the earth manageable for you, so traverse you through its tracts and enjoy of the sustenance which He furnishes ... (Q67: 14-15).*

7.1 Artificial Insemination in the Treatment of Infertility

Infertility or childlessness is defined as the failure of a couple to have a child after about a year of normal sexual intercourse without the use of contraceptives. This problem is increasing throughout the world, but there is evidence that it is more rampant in the developing countries. In many societies, infertility is a cause of emotional distress, disharmony and frequent divorce. Infertile women in certain cultures and communities are subjected to societal rebuke, intimidation and rejection. There are many methods of treating infertility depending on the causes; whether the problem is from the husband or the wife or both. Of these methods, artificial insemination stands out as a controversial one because of the moral and legal problems associated with it.

Artificial insemination[152] refers to the introduction of semen (containing sperms) into the vagina by means other than sexual intercourse (usually by suitably designed instruments or surgical procedures). Medically the main indications include inadequate insemination, azoospermia (no sperm in the semen), oligospermia (low sperm count or density), failure to ejaculate, retrograde (backward) ejaculation, impotence (either from lack of erection of the penis or premature ejaculation), castration, amputated penis, deleterious genes, etc. There are different methods of artificial insemination:

• Artificial Insemination Husband (AIR): In this method, the husband's semen is introduced into the reproductive organ of the wife.

• Artificial Insemination-Donor (Heterologous Insemination): This involves the introduction of sperm from a donor other than the husband into the wife. It is associated with a lot of legal and moral problems.

• In Vitro Fertilisation (IVF): This involves the collection of sperm from the husband and egg from the wife and fertilising in test tubes (that is why the resultant child is called a test tube baby), and then transferring the fertilised eggs (ova) into the womb of either the wife or another woman (surrogate motherhood). This method is resorted to if anatomical problems in the wife, which prevent an egg from reaching the uterine cavity (womb) cannot be treated surgically, or in a situation of the inability of sperms to reach the site of fertilisation (that is, within the fallopian tube).

---

152. The root of the word insemination is derived from the Latin word– seminare, that is, to sow, plant or beget and insemin(are); to implant or impregnate.

From the above, the remarkable contributions of science and the advances of modern developmental technology in solving the problems of man can be appreciated - notwithstanding the fact that Allah is the ultimate source of all knowledge. However, these advances raise as many questions or problems as they tend to solve. This is the scenario and challenge Zindani and his colleagues at the *Hay'at al-Ijaz al Ilmi* try, as an extension of similar works by scholars of Islarnisation of Knowledge programme, to combat or address. In page 12 of the book, *Human Development as Described in the Qur'an and sunnah,* Zindani *et al* summarised the situation:

> *How is society going to deal with the many moral, legal and ethical problems that can arise with embryos that have been produced by the many methods of artificial insemination? Children born of artificial insemination donor pose legal and moral problems of paternity. It may be legally proved that either the sperm donor or the husband or both are the fathers of the child. In the case of a test tube baby transferred into another woman's womb other than the supposed mother, both the women can as well claim motherhood of the child. How is society going to deal with the problems that can arise with embryos that have been produced by* **In vitro Fertilisation** *and then stored away in a freezer? What is to be done if the biological parents then die (as has already happened)? The products of such manipulation may well said to have five parents - the husband and the wife who donated the sperm and egg, the woman who receives the embryo and provides the*

uterine environment for *embryonic and fetal development of the child, and finally the man and woman who actually raise the child after birth. These are just few areas of a burgeoning concern. The physicians and scientists of today are, perhaps more than ever before, in need of the wisdom and counsel of scholars and religious leaders. It is therefore not surprising that we relook at our holy scriptures for help and enlightenment.*

With regards to the issue of permissibility, the Islamic view is clear on such matters and related issues.[153] If artificial insemination is between a husband and wife in their life time, it is permissible as long as the implantation is in the wife and the sperm is the husband's. Allah's Messenger (SAW) was reported as saying, "Whoever among you is able to help his brother should do so." Thus, Allah and His Messenger have enjoined relieving the distressed and benefiting humanity. As for artificial insemination involving a donor of semen other than the husband, it is outrightly prohibited in Islam. Both the Qur' an and Sunnah state that marriage is the only admissible way to having children, for it preserves and safeguards family ties, protects health and human values. Allah (SWT) says in the Qur'an:

And among His signs is this; that He created for you mates from among yourselves that you may dwell in tranquility with them and He has put love and mercy between your (hearts) (Q30:21).

153. Refer to the book *Human Development as Described in the Qur'an and Sunnah* which also cited the proceedings of an Islamic Conference held in Cairo in 1986 titled "Islam and Contemporary Medical Affairs.

He said further:

This day are (all) things good and pure made lawful unto you ... (lawful unto you in marriage) are (not only) chaste women who are believers, but chaste women among the People of the Book, revealed before your time. When you give them their due dowers, and desire chastity, not lewdness ... (Q5:5).

The renowned Islamic scholar Dr Yusuf Al-Qaradawi in his book, *The Lawful and The. Prohibited in Islam,* quoted Sheikh Shaltut as saying:

There is however no doubt that insemination by a donor other than the husband is a serious crime and a detestable offense, for the child born of such insemination incorporates in itself the result of adoption - the introduction of an alien element into the lineage in conjunction with the offense (similar to that) of adultery, which is abhorrent both to the divinely revealed laws and to upright human nature.

Thus, in Islam, children are to be born only of a husband and wife and of their family lineage. Those who are infertile either primarily (never had an issue) or had had offspring but ceased to produce others (secondary infertility), are reminded to recognise Allah as the source of cure for all afflictions, and at the same time embrace their destiny notwithstanding the efforts they make in securing a child by Allah's permission. The Qur'an states:

To Allah belongs the dominion of the heavens and the earth. He created what He wills, He bestows (children) male or female according to His will and He leaves barren (infertile) whom He wills, for He is full of knowledge and power (Q42:49-50).

According to the teachings of Islam, whatever Almighty Allah grants a person is a gift out of His abundant mercy and grace, and is neither a right nor an entitlement. However, this teaching is not an impediment to seeking for spiritual and material blessings or favours He provides for mankind. Hence, Islam permits other means and methods of the management of infertility, be it through medications, surgical procedures or lastly adoption.

The Qur'anic wisdom in granting the rights of polygamy and divorce, comes to our attention here, for it provides an infertile male the hope and succour of getting a child through a second wife as well as an infertile female with a similar chance through divorce and remarriage. However, divorce, of all the permissible things in Islam, is the most detested or hated by Allah *Subhanahu Wa Ta' alah*. Therefore, Islam more encouragingly recommends adoption. The adoption of a child is a meritorious act in the light of the Qur'an and Sunnah. The Prophet (SAW) was reported as saying:

I and the one who raises an orphan will be like these two in paradise. **And he pointed to his middle and index fingers with a slight gap between the two.**

Thus, an infertile couple can bring home an orphan or a foundling to rear, educate, feed, clothe, teach, love and protect as their own. If the infertile man or woman wishes such adopted child to benefit from his or her wealth, they may give him or her whatever they want during their life time, and may also bequeath to the adopted child up to one third (1/3) of their wealth before their death or by writing a will. However, Islam has prohibited the type of adoption which makes the adopted child a member of the family with all the rights of inheritance, the permissibility of mixing freely with the female members of the household, prohibition of marriage among them, bearing the family name and so on. On this account, the Qur'an states:

> *Nor has He (Allah) made your adopted sons your (real) sons, such is (only) your manner of speech by your mouths. But God tells you the truth and He shows the right way. Call them by the name of their fathers, that is juster in the sight of God. But if you know not their fathers name, call them your brothers in faith or your clients (Q33:4).*

Regardless of any method one chooses in seeking a solution to infertility, the basic approach is persistent prayers and supplication to God almighty as the source of cure for all afflictions and distress. This may not be unconnected with the psychological effect of infertility and the nature of seeking a solution to it, which in most cases is expensive, time consuming and discouraging. Hence, the Qur'an encourages infertile couples to earnestly and constantly offer their prayers to Allah for solution.

> *My Lord! Grant me from Yourself good offspring for You hear all prayers (Q3:38).*

And:

My Lord! Leave me not childless, though you
are the best of heirs (Q21 :89).[154]

The prayers above illustrate the Qur'anic account of the
flight of Prophet Zachariah (AS) who was childless at the
age of ninety-nine (99) while his wife was eighty-nine (89)
years old. Allah accepted their prayers and blessed them with
John the Baptist (AS). Another classical reference to infertility
in the Qur'an was the case of Prophet Abraham (AS) who in
his old age and with a wife who had attained menopause,
prayed thereof:

> *"My Lord! Grant me a righteous son." And We*
> *(answered his prayers and) gave him the good*
> *news of a gentle son (Q37: 100-101).*

Finally, we conclude that from the teachings of the Qur'
an and Sunnah, man is permitted in the words of the Prophet
(SAW) to "Seek for medical cure for Allah has not created a
disease without a cure." This cure involves all the means and
methods which do not go against human nature, morality
and divine laws. However, in all circumstances and times,
the principle of medicine in Islam stands; that Allah is the
source of all cure and everything is possible by His permission.
This concept and principle permeate all Islamic teachings,
and is summarised in the Prophet's prayer which he used to
recite before climbing animals as means of transport:

---

154. *See* also Qur'an 19:14-15, 3:38.

> *Glory be to Allah who has subjected these to our use, for we could never have accomplished this by ourselves and to Him must we turn back always for help.*

7.2 Abortion

Abortion is defined as the termination of pregnancy or premature expulsion of the product(s) of conception by any means usually before fetal viability.[155] Many terms are used for different types of abortion.[156] However, it is safe to say basically that abortion can be spontaneous or induced.

Spontaneous abortion (also called natural abortion or miscarriage) is an abortion that has not been induced artificially, it is usually an unwanted occurrence. In contrast, induced abortion is an abortion which is brought about intentionally by the use of instruments, medications or other devices, and is thus a wanted event. Again, induced abortion can be legal or illegal (that is, criminal). A legal abortion is one in which the indication for the abortion is purely medical, hence it is also called therapeutic abortion. A therapeutic abortion is an induced abortion performed because the continuation of the pregnancy might threaten the patient's life or seriously affect her health both physically (for example, underlying medical disorders such as heart disease, sickle cell disease, etc which may be complicated by allowing the pregnancy to grow), or mentally (for example, when the

---

155. Although the definition of viability varies from one environment to another, a human pregnancy of over a 20-week duration from the first day of the menstrual period, or a foetal weight of more than 500 grams, is usually termed viable in developed centre. In less developed areas, an average of 26 weeks is considered viable.
156. Other purely medical terminologies for abortion are incomplete, complete, missed, habitual, septic, induced, spontaneous, etc.

pregnancy is as a result of rape, incest, sex, abuse, etc), or when the continuation of the pregnancy is likely to result in the birth of a child with mental retardation or severe physical deformities that are not compatible with normal life. However, the discourse that follows refers to an abortion which is induced for reasons other than medical, mainly for social reasons. This is the type commonly referred to as illegal or criminal, depending on' the environment.

Islam's general approach to abortion is based on the right of both the child and the mother. Firstly, it is a divine injunction that no child becomes the cause of harm to the parents. Secondly, by implication the parents should reciprocate and cause the child no harm. According to these guidelines and, more specifically, one of the most inalienable rights of the child in Islam, is the right to life and equal life chances. The preservation of the child's life is the third commandment in Islam (Q6: 151, 17:31). While Islam permits preventing pregnancy for valid reasons, it does not allow tampering with the pregnancy once it occurs. Muslim jurists (scholars) agree unanimously that after the fetus is completely formed and has acquired a soul, abortion is prohibited under all circumstances, except to save the life of the mother. Sheikh Mahmond Shaltut stated in *his fatwa* concerning this issue as follows:

> For the mother is the origin of the fetus, moreover, she is established in life with duties and responsibilities and she is also a pillar of the family. It would not be possible to sacrifice her life for the life of a fetus, which has not yet acquired a personality and has no responsibilities or obligation.

Muslim scholars also attempt to grade the level of the prohibition of abortion based on the age of the pregnancy. Imam Ghazzali attempts to make a clear distinction:

> *Abortion is a crime against an existing being. Now existence has stages. The first stage is the settling of the semen in the womb and its mixing with the secretion of the woman. It is then ready to receive life, disturbing it is a crime. When it develops further and becomes a lump, aborting it is a greater crime. When it acquires a soul and its creation is completed, the crime becomes more grievous. The crime reaches its maximum seriousness when it is committed after it (the fetus) is separated from the mother alive.*

Therefore, the factors which determine the illegality or otherwise of abortion depends on the intentions and the prevailing situations, while the level of its illegality depends on the acquisition of spirit and the viability of the fetus. Statements from the Qur'an and Sunnah indicate that the spirit is acquired during the fetal period (Q23: 12-14, 15,29).[157] This indication signifies that the embryonic life prior to the fetal stage is of a different nature. Muslim scholars compared the nature of the embryonic period to the life of plants, since they are alive, but have no soul.[158]

The Qur'an further explains that after the attainment of definitive human form by the fetus, it then becomes viable and capable of sustaining life outside the uterus (womb) at

---

157. See *hadith* narrated by Abdullahi Ibn Mas'ud quoted earlier. "And God sends an angel to breath spirit unto the foetus…".
158. For details see chapter five on Research and Development.

about six (6) months of development, although the duration of normal pregnancy is 9 months (Q46: 15,2:233). This fact is in agreement with modern science, which puts 22 to 26 weeks as the period of viability of the fetus (which approximately equals 6 lunar months). Prior to the period of viability, the loss of the fetus or the termination of the pregnancy, is referred to as an abortion, since the fetus cannot survive. Such was the opinion of the 4th Caliph Ali bn Abi Talib (RA). This view was endorsed by the companions of the Prophet (SAW), as well as the Qur'anic commentators.

7.3 Family Planning

Family planning refers to the measures taken by couples to plan the number, timing and spacing of the children that they want in order to promote the health and welfare of the family group. Various methods are used in the attainment of this goal ranging from abstinence, contraceptive devices and pills to surgical procedures involving mainly the female group. The argument on the permissibility or prohibition of family planning was settled almost 15 centuries ago, for Allah (SWT) has stated in the Qur'an, "We are never unmindful of Our creation" (Q23: 17). However, recent attempts at introducing family planning services in traditional Muslim communities have given birth to both opponents and proponents of the act.

In general, family planning is in reality a long-time tradition and indeed part of the legacy of Islam. What are new are the modern methods which were unknown before. The contraceptive methods known and practised in the prophetic era were abstinence and *coitus interruptus* or *azl*, that is, withdrawal of the penis from the vagina before ejaculation. By analogous deduction *(qiyas)*, the Islamic ruling or position on *azl* apply also to other methods of contraception as long as the purpose is to prevent pregnancy within the limit allowed by Allah (SWT).

In earlier times, life was simpler and family life was less of a burden than it is today. Religious education was the norm through which the community augment the efforts of the parents whose child rearing responsibility was also shared by other members of the family. Under present circumstances, it is not easy for most parents to fulfill this obligation towards large families and the increasing demands of growing children. These obligations include:

- Maintenance and promotion of the physical (health) status of the family, particularly the mothers and children.

- Economic capability to support the family and safeguard the future of the children and provide separate sleeping areas for them.

- Cultural capability to give the child proper education and religious training.

- Time availability for children care and companionship, including verbal communication for stimulation of their intellectual development and promotion of parent-child affinity, love and intimacy.

Thus, family planning is not entirely a new concept since Islam has long ago prescribed measures, limitations and roles for parents with regards to family formation and childraising responsibilities. If the Islamic provisions are followed, parents will be able to raise children whom they will be able to honour their rights so that they become a source of joy to them, enrichment to their community and a support and defense for the nation. These rights, according to prophetic tradition, commence even before marriage and they can be condensed as follows:

- The right to life

- The right to genetic purity (legal marriages)

- The right to responsible parenthood

- The right to breast feeding, shelter, maintenance and support, including healthcare and nutrition

- The right to separate sleeping arrangements

- The right to future security

- The right to religious training and good upbringing

- The right to education and training in sport and self-defense

- The right to equitable treatment regardless of gender, etc

- The right that all funds used in their upbringing comes only from *halal* (legitimate) sources.

While Islam promotes marriage and procreation, it also made it clear that the desire for multitude should not be at the expense of qualitative parenthood as well as religious and mundane obligations. For instance, a child should be raised properly and in a manner that would bring honour to his parents, community and the Ummah. Islam frowns at miscreant behaviour, immorality, drug abuse, disobedience, neglect of religious practices, beggary and laziness. The Prophet (SAW) was reported by Amir bn Sa' ad bn Abi Waqqas in Sahih Bukhari saying:

Verily it is better for you to leave your offspring (heirs) wealthy than to leave them as poor beggars.

The Qur'an categorically cautions parents from seeing giving birth to so many children as an act that will solely please Allah and qualify them for special blessing.

It is not your wealth, nor your children that bring you nearer to Us, but only he who believes and does righteous deeds, as for such, there will be twofold reward for what they did, and they will reside in the high dwellings (paradise) in peace and security (Q 34:37).

As for the opponents of modern family planning, they also advance many arguments against the practice. Firstly, that multitude is ordained by religion since man's mission is to inhabit and develop the earth. The failure to achieve it is a deviation from the right path. In fact, the Prophet (SAW) has specifically encouraged all Muslims to be fruitful so that he can take pride of largest followership among the Prophets (PBUT) in the Day of Judgement. Fruitfulness is also the teaching of other revealed religions. For instance, in the Old Testament, speaking to Abraham (AS) concerning his son Ishmael, God said:

And I have blessed him, and will make him fruitful and will multiply him exceedingly (Genesis 17:20).

Secondly, that *al azl* or any practice that prevent conception is a minor form of infanticide, an act that has been categorically condemned and prohibited by Allah.

Kill not your children for fear of poverty. We shall provide (sustenance) for them as well as for you. Surely, the killing of them is a great sin (Q17:31).

And,

And the earth We have spread out and produced therein all kinds of things in due balance and We have provided therein means of sustenance for you and for those whose sustenance you are not responsible. And there is not a thing but its sources and treasures (inexhaustible) are with Us. But We only send down thereof in due and ascertainable measures. (Q15:19-21).

Deducing from the above, opponents of family planning are quick to condemn birth control practice based on the economic principle of limited resources and an over-increasing population (a theory propagated by Thomas Malthus, a famous English economist). This is because Allah is the creator and the provider for all His creatures. The problem is traceable or tied to corruption, greed, mismanagement and under utilisation or exploration of the natural resources which Allah has endowed mankind with. Further arguments against family planning by its opponent raised the allegation of conspiracy by the West to reduce the number of Muslims and diminish their power. On the doctrinal level, it is argued that family planning as a human intervention is against the spirit of *qadr* (predestination), *rizq* (provision) and *tawakkul* (reliance on Allah).

In view of the many arguments raised for or against family planning, it is essential for a believer to approach the issue with objectivity, fairness and *taqwa* (God's consciousness). In today's world, sheer population size has ceased to be the sole determinant of the political or military strength of any nation. The future of the Ummah, therefore, has more to do with quality, piety, solidarity and technological advancement than sheer numbers. A huge, overpopulated, weak, underdeveloped and fragmented nation held by shackles of poverty, disease, hunger, illiteracy, beggary and apathy cannot definitely be a subject of pride to anyone, let alone the Prophet! Many Qur'anic verses has laid emphasis on the multitude of quality and not merely of quantity (Q2:249, 5:100, 9:25, etc).

While mankind's goal on earth is to inhabit, populate and develop it, the supervening objective is to worship Allah as He should be worshipped (Q51:56). On the issue of equating contraception with infanticide, one needs to understand that the latter refers to the physical act of slaying a child or burying him or her alive (or forceful abortion of a viable foetus) - a detestable, condemnable and forbidden act. Whereas contraception is the mere act of preventing pregnancy and therefore involves no killing.

As to the issue of family planning originating from the West, it is not a basis for condemnation as the Prophet has said "knowledge is the lost property of the believer, he should pick it wherever he finds it." Moreover, one needs to appreciate the fact that family planning has its origin 15 centuries ago in the house of Islam.

On the issue of *qadr, rizq* and *tawakkul,* proponents of family planning also share the same beliefs. Contraception is only a means of attaining an objective, like planting of seeds on the ground; the results are in the hands of Allah. It can succeed or fail. Thus, reliance on Allah or belief in predestination and His ability to provide sustenance does not in all intents and purposes deny the Muslim the blessings and benefits of planning in his or her life. Moreover, such prospective planning is seen in other aspects of our lives; farming (cross-fertilisation, irrigation, dam construction and artificial rain), trade (investment), governance (budgets), education, animal husbandry (cross-breeding, castration, etc), artificial insemination, health (vaccines, prophylactic drugs, etc). Yet, no one considers such interventions as a negation of reliance on Allah.

In a *hadith* narrated by Anas bn Malik (RA) when an Arab Bedouin asked the Prophet (SAW) "Shall I leave my camel untied and seek Allah's protection on it, or should I tie it?" The Prophet answered, "Tie your camel and then depend upon Allah." This *hadith* emphasises the common concept of "God help those who help themselves."

In Islamic history, there is no instance of national policy that limits the number of children citizens of a state are allowed to produce per family. Most references to *azl* have more to do with specific individuals' cases rather than a general rule. There was an instance when the Prophet encouraged his companions to practise it during expeditions (obviously to avoid the burden and consequence of moving with weak and pregnant women during operations). However, at Medina during peace times he advised them to seek mutual consent of their wives before practising it.

Reconciling the various positions and opinions regarding the status of family planning, it is appreciable that the Sunnah has practically demonstrated its permissibility on genuine grounds. *Coitus interruptus* (withdrawal of the penis before ejaculation) is a type of contraception that was said to be in practice during the time of the Prophet (SAW). He came to know of it even among his companions, but he did not prohibit it. This is based on the *hadith* transmitted in both Sahih Bukhari and Muslim and narrated from the authority of Jubir (RA) who said, "We practised withdrawal *(azl)* during the time of the Messenger of Allah (SAW), while the Qur'an was being revealed. The Prophet came to know about it, but he did not prohibit it." In another version narrated by Abu Sa'id AI-Khudri (RA) in Sahih Bukhari transmission, the Prophet (SAW) was reported to have commented that, "Even then (that is, in spite of the *azl)* if Allah wishes to create a child no one can prevent it."

The statement of the Prophet (SAW) above implies that despite the employment of *coitus interruptus,* a drop of semen containing sperm might be deposited in the vagina without one's awareness, and if Allah so wishes, it will result in conception. Thus, while Islam regards it as excessive and a transgression of bounds by man to use crude methods on a wider scale to limit population based on "population-explosion," socio-economic breakdown or whatever reasons, it does not deny man the benefits of planning his society using means and methods acceptable to Allah. Consequently, the following are a few examples of the circumstances under which family planning services may be permissible:

- **Obstetric and gynaecological conditions:** for example, a woman with vesico vaginal fistula (VVF), following a prolonged obstructed labour if delivered by surgical intervention (caesarian section) will benefit from family planning to avoid the hazards or risks of another pregnancy within a short time. Other conditions are grand multiparity, advanced age (above 44 years), contracted or small pelvis, recurrent or habitual abortion (successive miscarriages), difficult and operative deliveries and other high-risk pregnancies.

- **Medical conditions:** Women with sickle cell disease (tend to have increased incidence of morbidity and death with each successive pregnancy), diabetes mellitus (tend to have large babies during pregnancy which predisposes them to prolonged and obstructed labour), and certain blood group incompatibility between the mother and the offspring. Other medical conditions include women with HIV infection or AIDS, hypertension, cardiovascular disorders, recurrent congenital anomalies, etc.

- **Maternal and Child health:** Short intervals between two pregnancies and deliveries have been shown to have adverse effects on both the elder and the younger baby. The elder child is predisposed to protein energy malnutrition (murasmus, kwashiorkor or underweight), child abuse or neglect, poor mental development, failure to thrive, stunted growth, etc. Studies have also shown that infants born 12 months or less after previous pregnancies have a slightly increased risk of morbidity and neonatal death. In general, adequate child spacing (2-3 years) gives the mother enough time to recover both physically and mentally from her previous pregnancy. She will be able to replenish her nutritional reserves which will prevent the development of maternal depletion syndrome (a serious medical disorder which affects the mother and consequently the child).

- **Other Conditions (Vnspecified)**[159]

It is reported in an authentic tradition[160] that in a gathering at which Umar (RA) was present, someone said that *coitus interruptus* was a minor form of burying a child alive, but Ali bn Abi Talib (RA) then responded. "This is not so before the completion of seven stages, being a product of the earth, then a drop of semen, then a clot, then a lump of tissue, then bones, then bones clothed with flesh, which then become

---

159. It has been deduced by scholars through qiyas that there may be reasons other than health matters for which a couple can practice contraception. Such reasons may be occupational (military engagement), educational pursuit, scholarship, itinerancy, trade, burdens of leadership, disasters, economic hardship on the family, disputes, etc.
160. Cited by Al-Qaradawi in his book *"The Lawful and The Prohibited in Islam."*

another creature."[161] On the basis of this *hadith,* scholars consider *fatwa* on contraception or abortion based on the stages they are practised. Some Muslim scholars commenting on the verse "Kill not your children," inferred that the command does not necessarily refer to contraception, but to the acts of burying the child alive as practised by Arabs during the *jahiliyyah (pre-Islamic)* period, and may include our modern day abortion for such purposes. This is because in contraception, the conception is altogether prevented and does not even involve a disturbance to the product of conception, not to talk of relating it to murder.

Therefore, family planning services can be utilised based on the validity of the reasons. However, the applicability of the methods depends on an individual's circumstances and intentions, for it may be permissible to one couple and prohibited to another. The methods are also invariably based on individual's need. Whatever the circumstances and intentions, Allah is the best judge.

> *Mothers shall breast feed their children for two whole years for him who wishes the sucking to be completed. None shall be charged with more than one can bear. A mother should not be allowed to suffer on account of her child, nor should a father on account of his child ... have fear of Allah and know that He is cognisant of all your actions. (Q2:233).*

---

161. It is as a result of these scientific deductions from the Qur'an and Sunnah by the Suhabah (Companions of the Prophet) that enabled Caliph Umar (RA) to lay down a legal ruling that delivery of a 26 week old pregnancy after marriage is legitimate and acceptable.

7.4 HIV Infection and AIDS

The term Acquired Immune Deficiency Syndrome (AIDS) describes the later stage of infection by the Human Immunodeficiency Virus (HIV) of which two types are known - I and II. The cardinal feature of the disease is suppression (weakening) of the immunity (defense mechanisms) of the human body, thereby predisposing the affected person to a variety of clinical disorders including infections and malignancies (cancers). AIDS today is one of the greatest threats to the existence of mankind. It has spared no community, country or continent. The World Health Organisation (WHO), in a series of reports, admits that there is no definite cure against HIV infection or AIDS, and that the best option or alternative is the prevention of its transmission. In spite of the knowledge of its transmission, of which sexual contact carries the highest percentage, and the scientific methods of its prevention, AIDS today continues alarmingly to be on the rampage every hour of the day. Without doubt, HIV / AIDS infection provides one of the greatest challenges to the medical community, researchers and scientists of the world.

AIDS entered the world's consciousness and become part of the vocabulary of the human soul, as a result of a dawning awareness of the advent of a strange or new disease. It was first reported in 1981. Since then, the cumulative number of HIV infected or AIDS cases reported to the World Health Organisation has been on the increase. According to the Joint United Nations Programme on HIV/AIDS (UNAIDS), the number of adults currently infected with HIV throughout the world is about forty (40) million, out of which eight to twenty-four (8-24) million adults will develop AIDS by the end of the century. No wonder, Albert Camus in "Evolution of a Pandemic" was quoted as saying:

*The plague (of AIDS) had swallowed up
everything and everyone. No longer were there
individual destinies, only a collective destiny,
made up of the plague and the etnotions shared
by all. The strongest of these emotions was the
sense of exile and of deprivation, with all the
crosscurrents of revolt and fear set up by these.*[162]

However, this calamity was foretold about fourteen (14)
centuries ago. The Qur'an states:

*Whatever misfortune happens to you, is because
of the things your hands have wrought, and for
many. He grants forgiveness (Q42:30).*

The Prophet (SAW) was also reported in Sunan Ibn Majah
as saying:

*Lewdness has never prevailed among a nation
until it becomes an open practice, then epidemic
diseases and pain unknown to their ancestors
will appear among them.*

Thus, in accordance with the above Qur'anic verse and
the *hadith* of the Prophet (SAW), vices such as homosexuality,
bisexuality, illegal heterosexuality (fornication and adultery)
are open invitations to human immunodeficiency virus (HIV)
(regardless of the controversies surrounding its origin and so
on) and other sexually transmitted diseases. It should also be
made clear that Islam considers HIV infection and AIDS and
indeed any type of calamity or disaster as part of the "tests
and trials of life" which can afflict both the righteous, and

---

162.   *See HIV and AIDS: A Strategy for Nursing Care* by Pratt, R, J. pp. 10-220.

the profligate – whence a calamity befall a nation, it afflicts all, for everyone has a stake in it. Hence, it is not exclusively a disease of sinners, since it has no exemption for saints, children and the innocent.

As far as Islam is concerned, the best alternative for man is that, he must recognise the existence of Allah and His complete Lordship. It is He alone who possesses sovereignty and the right to ordain a path for mankind. About 1400 years ago the holy Qur' an came with a legislation that protects man and guards him from disasters (such as AIDS):

> *And come not near adultery for it is an indecent (deed) and an evil way (Q17:32).*

> *Let those who find not the means of marriage keep themselves chaste until Allah gives them means out of His Grace (Q24:33).*

On the other hand, as for those who can afford marriage, Islam also encourages marrying faithful partners, which is one of the cardinal preventive measures against my transmission.

> *Marry those among you who are single, or the virtuous ones ... (Q24:32).*

The Qur' an made it a prohibition for a believer to marry an adulterer or adulteress (Q24:3, 24:26). Islam places so much emphasis on faithful partnership among couples that it even allows Muslims to marry virtuous women among non-Muslims in preference to unchaste women among Muslims, because of the foreseen danger associated with the latter.

> *Lawful unto you in marriage are (not only)*
> *chaste women who are believers, but chaste*
> *women among the People of the Book (Jews and*
> *Christians) (Q5:5).*

In order to accommodate all men of varying social inclinations, physiology, sexual appetite and to avoid extramarital sex, Islam permits (not command) marrying an additional wife or wives, not exceeding a maximum of four (Q4:3). In order to safeguard the right of both husband and wife against unfaithfulness, Islam guarantees the freedom of an amicable dissolution of the marriage through divorce (Q2:228, 4:35). This will enable both parties to explore, alternatively, the happiness, compassion, peace and security of marital life. However, if faithfulness is not adhered to in marriage, polygamy (and indeed monogamy) becomes a window for acquiring sexually transmitted infections, including HIV/AIDS.

Several studies have shown that sexual intercourse during menstruation carries a high risk of HIV transmission in a HIV infected woman as well as other sexually transmitted diseases (syphilis, gonorrhoea, chlamydia, chanroid, pelvic inflammatory disease, trachomoniasis, etc).

This may be one of the reasons why Islam forbids it:

> *Keep away from women in their menstrual*
> *periods and do not approach them until they*
> *are clean (Q2:222).*

Generally with regard to decency and sexual morality, Allah commanded His Prophet (SAW) to proclaim His message to the world.

> *And say to the believing women that they should guard their chastity (Q24:31).*

And:

> *Successful indeed are the believers (male or female) ... who guard their modesty (Q23: 1 and 5).*

Thus, a believer must guard himself or herself against every kind of illegitimate sex, abuse, perversion or deviation. The new psychology associated with the name of Freud has traced many hidden motives to sex, and it is common knowledge that a man's refinement or degradation may be measured by the hidden workings of his or her sexual instincts.[163] That is why Islam recognises and harnesses instincts for the good of man in this world and the next.

It is in line with this guiding principle of Islam that Muslim medical scientists and health professionals adopt an Islamic moral value-based approach to HIV/AIDS prevention and control. One such example is from the activities of the Islamic Medical Association of Uganda (IMAU), a Non-Governmental Organisation, which has succeeded in integrating Islamic religious values and wisdom with scientific medical information on HIV/AIDS. This approach has been recognised internationally by the joint United Nations Programme on HIV/AIDS (UNAIDS) in their latest publication on the best practice collection in the combat against AIDS.

There is ample scientific evidence that this approach (of utili sing Islamic principles and teachings and scientific information to promote behaviours that prevent and control

---

163. Sigmund Freud (1856-1939) an Austrian psychiatrist and founder of classical psychoanalysis, was credited with making a remarkable contribution in the psychology of sex and instincts.

HIV infection) proves successful in several communities where applied. According to a case-control study conducted in a rural Uganda community on the "Risk for HIV- I infection in Adults," "there is a reduction in the risk of infection among Muslims in comparison with non-Muslims," and the researchers suggests that "the protective effect of male circumcision and difference in lifestyles may account for this disparity."

Another related study conducted in Uganda by researchers from the Medical Research Council (UK) programme on AIDS in Uganda and the Uganda Virus Research Institute, reveals that "Muslims have significantly lower rates of HIV infection (6.1 %) in comparison with non-Muslims (27.4%)". The researchers further stated that:

> *The findings that Muslims are at a decreased risk compared with non-Muslims is consistent with those from other studies, including another Uganda population. Two studies of African countries have assessed the correlation between the estimates of the population to that of the male population who have been circumcised and zero-prevalence rates of HIV/AIDS; both studies support the hypothesis that lack of circumcision is a risk factor. In our study, since male circumcision in this population is not practised outside the Muslim community, it is possible that this difference, which is found not only in men but also in women, may be due to the possible protective effect of circumcision to both men and their partners.*

However, apart from circumcision, other factors related to Muslims were considered to explain the reduced rate of

HIV transmission. These include the protective effect of marriage in the older age group (above 25 years), marital faithfulness and the avoidance of sexual intercourse during menstruation. In line with this development, the Islamic Medical Association of Uganda under the leadership of Dr Magid Kagimu in collaboration with other agencies and bodies interested in the combat against AIDS, have introduced many pioneering initiatives and innovative approaches to HIV prevention based on the Islamic teachings in the Qur' an and Sunnah. Thus, it is high time Muslim health professionals and health workers adopt this strategy and incorporate the Islamic values and ethics in the *Jihad* (struggle) against HIV/AIDS infection.

The Hope for Cure

As far as Islam is concerned, God is Merciful and Compassionate. By changing our sexual attitude and exploring other natural bounties through research and technology, a definite cure for HIV or AIDS infection is not out of reach. The Prophet (SAW), inspired by divine knowledge, has said:

> *Allah has never brought a disease without providing a cure, when the right medicine strikes the disease it will be cured by the will of Allah.*[164]

The Qur' an confirms that:

> *Man can have nothing but what he strives for. That (the fruit of) his striving will soon come in sight. Then will he be re-warded with a reward complete (Q53:39-44).*

---

164. Reported from Abubakar (RA) in Sahih Muslim.

Thus, from the Qur'an and Sunnah, Muslims, and humanity in general, are encouraged to continue along the path of research to explore the cure for all ailments afflicting man. Surely the "right medicine" mentioned by the Prophet will one day be found by Allah's permission.

> *Never give up hope of Allah's soothing mercy; truly no one despairs of Allah's mercy except those who have no faith (Q12:87).*

7.5 Immunisation and Prophylaxis

Immunisation is the process of creating or improving the body's resistance to infection by artificial means. The process involves the administration or injection of suspensions or modified products of infectious agents used directly as antigens, which, when introduced into the body, stimulate the production of antibodies (natural agents of body defence against microbial invasion) against a specific disease. Prophylaxis involves the usage of certain drugs purposely to serve as protective measures against an impending disease. The Qur'an states:

> *Against them (your enemies) make ready your strength to the utmost of your power ... (Q8:60).*

And:

> *... and let them take their precautions and their arms (Q4: 102).*

In an authentic narration by Abu Hurairah (RA), the Messenger of Allah (SAW) said:

Whosoever eats honey (at least) three times every week will meet with no great affliction.

It is also reported in Sahih Bukhari from the authority of Sai'd Thn Abi Waqas (RA) that the Messenger of Allah (SAW) said:

Whoever takes seven dates every morning, he will be protected from the effect of poison and sorcery.

From the above statements of the Qur'an and the *ahadith*, Muslim scholars drew a conclusion on the permissibility of immunisation and prophylaxis because it was practised by the Prophet (SAW). They also make an analogy from the Qur'anic narration of the story of Joseph (AS) who in anticipation of a famine (which he prophesied to the Egyptian king) kept ample reserves of food in order to alleviate the impending calamity (Q12:55). The narrated tradition of the Prophet (SAW) during the battle of the trench *(Khandaq)* provides also a similar analogy when the Prophet and his companions dug a protective trench round the town of Madina against the approaching unmatchable army of their invaders.

However, some scholars of Islam consider any act of taking medicine before an illness as a prohibition because it connotes an act of ascribing a cure or protection to the drug or substance taken. They based their arguments on the Qur'anic verse: "If Allah touches you with affliction none can remove it but He. He hath power over all things" (Q6: 17).

Furthermore, condensing the opinions of many Muslim scholars and taking into consideration the spirit of Islam in all its teachings and the statement of the Prophet. (SAW),

"Whoever among you is able to help his brother should do so," one can infer that prophylactic treatment and immunisation against certain diseases is permissible in the light of the Qur'an and Sunnah. Nevertheless, we add that, as in all other medications and efforts to provide a cure or treatment, Islam enjoins man to have a firm belief *(iman)* in Allah as the source of all cures and remedies. This is one of the basic principles of Islamic medicine as opposed to secular medicine, which disowns God and His control over the mechanisms of disease and cure.

CHAPTER EIGHT

Necessity Dictates Exception

8.1 Doctors Examining Patients of the Opposite Sex

It is the standard routine in medical practice for doctors to examine their patients regardless of the difference in the sexes. On many occasions, some Muslim patients refuse to be examined by a male or female doctor, insisting that the examining doctor must be of their sex. In most cases, this is not possible because of the staggering difference in the proportion of male doctors to the few female doctors. It is observed that a majority of patients resent being stripped naked, and in addition female patients in most cases refuse vaginal or anal examination (which are common procedures in clinical assessment in the hospitals).

These are serious issues which need to be clarified. The truth is that Islam is not oblivious to the exigencies of life and their magnitude, nor to human weaknesses and the capacity to face them. It permits the Muslim under the compulsion of necessity to eat prohibited food in quantities sufficient to remove the necessity and save life. In the Qur'anic context, after listing the prohibited foods in the form of dead animals, blood and pork, God the Almighty says:

But if one is compelled by necessity neither craving (it) nor transgressing, there is no sin on him; indeed Allah is forgiving, Merciful (Q2: 173).

This is repeated in about four places in the Qur'an after each mention of the prohibited foods. On the basis of these and similar verses of the Qur'an, Islamic scholars formulated an important principle, namely, that "necessity removes restrictions." In permitting the use of the *haram* or its applicability under necessity - Islam is true to its spirit and general principles. This spirit, which we find permeating its laws, is to make life easy and not oppressive for human beings.

Allah desires ease for you and He does not desire hardship for you (Q2: 185).[165]

The Messenger of Allah also clarifies further: "He among you who sees anything wrong should rectify it (according to the degree of his faith) with his hands (power), or tongue (preaching), or his heart (that is, inward resentment)."[166] Furthermore, the Prophet (SAW) stated, "God Almighty has forgiven my followers their actions based on error, ignorance or under compulsion or necessity." [167]

Imam As-Suyuti in his *Tibbi Nabawi* reported that, "Imam Ahmed says that it is *halal* for a physician to examine a woman, even though they are not related, whenever it is

---

165. *See* also Qur'an 2:178, 4:28, 5:6 etc.
166. From Abu Sa'id Al-Khudri in Sahih Muslim.
167. From Ibu Abbas in Sunan Ibn Majah.

necessary to do so, and including the private parts." This was also the *fatwa* of Al-Maruzi (in !lis book of *hadith*), Al-Athram and Isma'il. Similarly, it is *halal* for a woman to look at the private parts of a man in a case of necessity. Harab stated this in his collection of *hadith*.

Thus, from the above, Islam permits a Muslim male or female to be examined by a medical doctor of the opposite sex, whether Muslim or non-Muslim as the circumstances demand. However, with patience, hardwork and dedication, the problem would be solved in the long run if more females and more Muslims join the medical profession. Imam AI-Ghazzali in his book, *Ihya'u ulumiddin (Revivification of Religious sciences)*, mentioned that, "Members of the Muslim community are collectively sinful before Allah (SWT), if they do not have enough doctors to cure or look after their patients." The Qur'an is our best reminder!

> *Man can have nothing except what he strives for (Q53:39).*

> *And strive in His cause as you ought to strive, (with sincerity and under discipline). He has chosen you (as Muslims), and has imposed no difficulties on you in religion ... (Q22:78).*

And:

> *Go you forth and strive and struggle with your goods and persons. That is best for you if you (but) knew (Q9:4l).*

Thus, the challenge is ours!

8.2 Females in Medical Practice

Islam recognises the right of women in equality with men in so far as it is compatible with the nature of the two sexes. The Qur'an states:

> And their Lord accepted their prayers (saying):
> 'Never will I suffer to be lost the work of any of
> you – whether male or female (Q3: 195).

The Qur' an further states:

> To men is the benefit of what they earn and to
> women what they earn (Q4:32).

In another verse the Qur'an states:

> And women shall have rights similar to the
> right against men according to what is equitable,
> but men have a degree over them (Q2:228).

It is related in Sahib Bukhari that the Messenger of Allah (SAW) was reported by Aisha (RA) as saying, "O women! You have been allowed by Allah to go out for your needs." It is also reported by Bukhari, Muslim and others, that in an authentic narration from Sahl Thn Sa' ad Al-Ansari, the Prophet (SAW) and his companions were served with wedding food by the wife of their post, Abu U sayd AI-Sa' ad, and the Prophet (SAW) did not prohibit that. It is reported in many traditions that women during the time of the Prophet (SAW) participated in taking care of the sick and the wounded and by removing the wounded and the slain from the battlefield, and even taking part in the actual fighting, when the occasion arose or the situation called for it.

It is transmitted in Sahib Muslim that Ummu 'Atiyya (RA) said, "We travelled with the Prophet (SAW) on seven expeditions. I travelled at the rear with the baggage. I prepared their food and I treated the sick and the wounded." It was also reported from the authority of Anas (RA) that, "The Prophet (SAW) went on an expedition, and he took Ummu Salama (his wife) with him, and with her came some of the women folk of the *Ansar.* They used to take the drinking water around, and they used to treat the wounded." This *hadith* has been transmitted by Muslim.

It was narrated by Sahal bn Sa'ad that the Prophet's daughter, Fatima (RA), then aged 19 or 20 years, lovingly nursed her father's wounds at the battle of Uhud (A.H 3). It was also narrated that Rufaida nursed Sa'ad Ibn Mu'azu's wounds at the siege of Madina by the confederate tribes (A.H 5). In the Khaibar expedition (A.H. 7), Muslim women also went out from Madina for nursing services. Several traditions have shown that the ladies of the Prophet's household engaged themselves in social work and that of instruction for the Muslim women, and that Muslim women were being trained more and more in community service. In fact, two of the wives of the Prophet (SAW), Zainab bint Khuzaimat (nicknamed "mother of the poor" for her generosity) and Zainab bint Jahsh (RA), worked for the poor, for whom they provided for from the proceeds of their manual work, as they were skilful in leather work. Hence, all the wives of the Prophet in their esteemed position did not live idle lives. They worked and assisted as mothers of the *Ummah,* and even helped the Prophet in his duties of leadership.

Thus, there is nothing wrong, other than reward and benefit, for Muslim women to be encouraged to study medicine as well as other branches of knowledge and offer health services among others to their community.[168] The most important thing is that the woman must conduct herself according to Islamic teachings (especially in terms of dressing and behaviour).

8.3 Seeking Health Services from Non-Muslims

There is no harm done if Muslims at either the governmental or private level seek help from non-Muslims in their worldly affairs, for example, medical services, industry, agriculture, the military, etc.

Allah forbids you not, with regard to those who fight you not for (your) faith nor drive you out of your homes, for dealing kindly and justly with them. For Allah loveth those who are just (Q60:8).[169]

The Prophet (SAW) demonstrated this teaching when he employed Abdullahi Thn Uraiqit, a polytheist, to be his guide

---

168. Here again, attention is drawn to the clear distinction between an Islam culture and the culture of individual Muslim communities. Hence, it is not surprising to find people attitudes or behaviour of some Muslim to Islam. Though, ideally all Muslims are supposed to behave and act islamically, in some cases it is not so. There are some who out of ignorance or weakness adopt certain attitudes which are not essentially derived from Islamic sources, but from cultural norms of their forefathers. In many places in the Qur'an Allah condemns such attitudes.

Therefore, those Muslims who in name of *purdah*, absolutely disallow their wives or daughters from seeking for knowledge, securing gainful employment, or preventing them from seeking medical services for their ailments, should be sadly and regretfully considered in this context. (*see* Q2:170, 26:24, etc).

169. *See* also Qur'an 5:82

on his flight from Mecca to Medina. He also sought help from Jews in issues of common national interest. Some early Muslim leaders among the Prophet's companions used to employ Christians and Jews as interpreters in judicial matters or settling disputes (even when such cases were conducted in the mosques).[170] It is related by Aisha (RA) in authentic narration, that:

> *The Prophet (SAW) had many illnesses during which several physicians, both Arab and non-Arab, used to come and sit next to him and treat him.*

This *hadith* further demonstrates that health services among people recognise no barrier since it is a matter of utmost necessity.

The condition for seeking help from a non-Muslim is that he or she must be trustworthy and knowledgeable in his or her field. At the same time it is of course extremely desirable that Muslims become self-sufficient.

8.4   The Use of Cadavers (Dead Bodies) for Medical Training

The Prophet (SAW) was reported as saying, "Whoever relieves a believer of one of the tragedies of this life, Allah will

---

170. It must be pointed out that the enmity or hatred referred to in certain place in the Qur'an between Muslims and non- muslims in most cases are specific to place, time and people. It does not in general terms implies that Muslim see non-Muslims as perpetual enemies. The Qur'an has it clear that the detestation is for evil not for men as such, so long as there is a chance for any repentance. Thus, it is mischievous for scholar (Muslim or non- Muslim) to make outright generalization in verses which come with specifica-tion, and in exclusion of other verses which shed more light and give more meaning to such verses in any given circumstances (*see* Qur'an 9:14, 8:32, 48:22;60:1-9, 22:39, 2:246, 2:216, 2:244).

relieve him of one of the calamities of the Day of Resurrection."[171] In another *hadith* narrated by Jabir in Sahih Muslim, the Prophet (SAW) also said, "Whoever among you is able to help his brother should do so." The Qur'an enjoins man to see things in the light of reality and practical life. It states:

> *On the earth are signs for those of assured faith.*
> *As also in your own selves: will you not then*
> *observe? (Q51:21).*

And:

> *We created man of the best structure (Q95:4)*

The Prophet (SAW) said, "Knowledge is the lost property of the believer he should pick it wherever he sees it." In another place the Prophet (SAW) was reported as saying "Seeking for knowledge is obligatory on every Muslim (male or female)."

Thus, if seeking for knowledge entails studying the cadaver (dead body) at the laboratory, then it becomes permissible based on the rule of necessity.[172] The same rule may also apply to the post-humous examination of dead bodies (autopsy) by pathologists in order to find the real cause of death, either for research or legal purposes. However, all manner of dealing with the human body even while alive (in terms of respect, honour, privacy and dignity) should be observed as much as possible. Islam teaches that every human being has dignity and position, regardless of his or her beliefs.

---

171. Narrated by Abu Hurairah in Sahih Muslim.
172. This is the opinion and *fatwa* of the majority of Al-Azhar scholars (see *NaqlulA' ada' i Baynal Dibbi Waddeeni* of Sheikh Mustapha Az-Zahbi. Darul Hahith Publishers. Cairo, Egypt.

It is reported in an authentic narration that: "Once a funeral procession passed by the Prophet and he stood up. Thereupon someone remarked, "O Messenger of Allah, it is the funeral of a Jew." The Prophet (SAW) then replied, "Was he not a soul?"

In many places in the holy Qur'an, Allah has drawn our attention to the anatomy of His creation as a demonstration of His wisdom and knowledge, and He also challenged humankind to recapitulate and reflect over such honours and bounties:

> *Do they not look at the camels, how they are created? And at the sky, how it is raised high? And at the mountains, how they are fixed firm? And at the earth, how it is spread out? (Q88: 17-20).*

On human anatomy, the Qur'an states:

> *Does man think that We cannot assemble his bones? Nay, We are able to put together in perfect order the very tips of his fingers*[173] *(Q75:3-4).*

> *Have We not made for man a pair of eyes? And a tongue, and a pair of lips? (Q90:8-9).*

And:

> *Glorify the name of your Guardian Lord, Most High, who hath created, and further given order and proportion (Q87: 1-2).*

---

173. As a point fact, medical scientists, particularly anatomists are in the best position to appreciate this Qur'anic verse - a pointer to the delicate arrangement of the structure of the extrinsic and intrinsic muscles (lumbricals, interossei, thenar, hypothenar, etc) the nerves, capillaries, bones and multiple joints.

On mutation and anatomical variation:

> *Praise be to Allah... , He adds to creation as He pleases; for Allah has power over all things. What Allah out of His mercy doth bestow on mankind none can withhold (and) what He doth withhold none can grant apart from Him, and He is the exalted in power, full of wisdom (Q35: 1-2).*

On the field of paediatrics and geriatrics:

> *It is Allah Who created you in a state of (helpless) weakness then gave (you) strength after weakness and a hoary head; He creates whatever He wills; and it is He who hath all knowledge and power (Q30:54).*

And:

> *And Allah has created you and then He will cause you to die; and of you there are some who are sent back to senility, so that they know nothing after having known (much). Truly Allah is All-Knowing, All-Powerful (Q16:70).*

Hence, the scientific study of the human creature for the spiritual and physical benefits of man may, by implication, be an extension of the Qur'anic statement:

> *Soon We will show them Our signs in the horizons of the earth and in themselves until it becomes manifest to them that this is the truth (Q4.1 :53).*

Therefore, Islam encourages education and learning for the benefit of man, and this was the very first teaching of the divine message of Allah. Besides, the Qur'an enjoins man to observe, study, think and contemplate over the phenomena of nature, what the Qur' an calls *Ayat I Allah*.[174]

8.5 Treating Illnesses with Prohibited Substances or Means

There is difference of opinion among Muslim scholars concerning whether some prohibited substances or food can be used as medicine. Those who argue that there is sufficient and authentic evidence in the Prophet's Sunnah to indicate the prohibition of using *haram* substances (such as wine or insulin extracted from pig) as medicine, cited the Prophet's statement, "Assuredly Allah has not made a cure for your sicknesses in what he has prohibited to you."[175]

Other scholars consider the need for medicine equal to that of food, as both are necessary for preserving life. They argued in support of their position that prohibited food substances may be used as medicine because the Prophet (SAW) himself allowed AbdulRahman Thn Awf and Zubair Thn AI-Awwam to wear silk shirts (in spite of its prohibition ordinarily) because they were suffering from scabies and had itching when they wore cotton and woollen shirts.[176]

Dr Yusuf AI-Qaradawi is of the opinion that the latter view is close to the spirit of Islam which in all its legislation and teaching, is concerned with the preservation of human life. However, taking medicine containing some *haram* substance is permissible under the following conditions:

---

174. Meaning the signs of God, that is, phenomena pointing to the creator.
175. From Ibn Mas'ud (RA) in Sahih Bukhari transmission.
176. From Qnas (RA) in the *Sahah* collection.

- The patient's life is endangered if he does not take the medicine.

- No alternative or substitute medication made from entirely *halal* sources is available.

- The medication is preferably prescribed by a physician who is knowledgeable and God-conscious.

It is in this light we consider blood transfusion and organ donation or transplantation, which though ordinarily prohibited, yet necessity has made permissible. Many scholars have outrightly pointed out the prohibition of selling a part or whole of the human body, whether dead or alive, for whatever purpose. But present day circumstances and the reality of the practical life has made these practices and attitudes acceptable throughout the Muslim world.[177] This again is based on the already established Islamic guiding spirit and the concept of "necessity removes restrictions."[178]

8.6   Medication and Instrumentation for the Fasting Patients

Fasting means abstaining from food, drink and legitimate sexual intercourse from dawn until sunset. Fasting during the month of Ramadan (which is the ninth month in the Islamic calendar) is a fundamental religious obligation.

---

177. In contrast, some Christian sects and denomination such as the Jehovah Witnesses without any compromise condemn and reject blood transfusion under ALL circumstances. They do not consider the fact on ground that medical facilities are not equitably distributed in the world. Thus, while bloodless surgery may be possible in one community it may not be in another even at a time of dire hard emergency!

178. The Prophet (SAW) was reported to have said; "Extreme necessity srenders *Haram (unlawful)* as *Halal* (permissible)."

Fasting in any month other than Ramadan is considered supererogatory or optional, except otherwise indicated as specific provision. According to the teachings of Islam, fasting is primarily a spiritual discipline. However, there are also other benefits - moral, economic, legal, educational and medical among others associated with the practice.

The issue of treating patients observing the fast (compulsory or optional) in many cases constitutes a potential problem in medical practice. Many uninformed Muslim patients refuse taking any medication or even examination by doctors on the ground that such an act will nullify their fasting. This is absurd, ridiculous and far from being a clear understanding of the letter and spirit of Islam. The Qur'an states categorically:

> *O ye who believe! Fasting is prescribed to you as it was prescribed to those who were before you ..., for a fixed number of days; but if any of you is ill or on a journey, the prescribed number should be made up from days later (Q2: 183-184).*

It is narrated by Yahya that he heard Imam Malik saying:

> *What I have heard from the people of knowledge is that, 'If a man succumbs to an illness which makes fasting difficult for him and exhausts him and wears him out, he can break his fast. This is the same as with a sick person in the salat (prayer), who finds standing to be too difficult and exhausting and he prays sitting – this is Allah's ease'.*

Therefore, fasting in Islam is not for self-torture, but for spiritual and physical elevation of man. The verse quoted above clearly exempts the sick person from observing the fast. Muslim scholars drawing conclusion from the above and related Qur'anic verses and *hadith,* said a Muslim who refuses medication in order to preserve his or her fasting and then dies as a result of the illness is guilty of committing suicide. In fact, the Islamic provision on fasting is very practicable and simple; it exempts even those who experience difficulty in observing fasting (for example, the aged, pregnant women, lactating mothers, travellers, etc.[179] The Qur'an states:

For those who can do it (fasting) with hardship, is a ransom, the feeding of one who is indigent (Q2: 184).

In order to emphasise the mercy of God and the dynamism of Islam, the Qur'an repeated its concessions or exemptions on fasting for the sick.

But if anyone is ill, the prescribed period (for fasting) should be made up by later days. Allah intends every facility for you; He does not want to put you to difficulties ... In that He has guided you and perchance, you shall be grateful (Q2:185).

Facilitation is the natural Sunnah recommended to the Prophet (SAW) by Allah in order to make His *deen* attractive. It is categorically made clear and agreed by all scholars that even when the statement of Allal) is clear-cut on prohibition

179.   For details see *The Book of Fasting* by Sheikh Ahmed Lemu, pp. 6-29.

or otherwise of a particular thing, the rule of facilitation in cases of utmost necessity shall prevail. This is neither a contradiction nor a negation of the divine injunction, but an extension of its wisdom and mercy. Therefore, in conclusion, Islam permits patients to seek for all forms of medical services while fasting, and if the need arises to break the fast or forfeit it altogether on account of the illness.

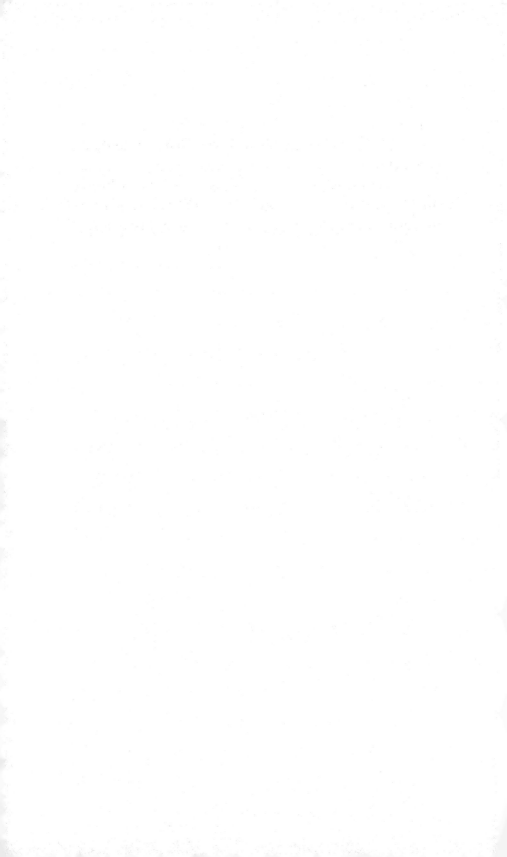

CHAPTER NINE

Muslims and the Practice of Medicine

9.1 Historical Background

In observation of Allah's injunctions, the world of Islam, from the time of the Prophet (SAW) and the four (4) rightly-guided Caliphs (RA)[180] through the ages, has used scientific knowledge contained in the Qur'an for the organisation, growth and development of their societies. This trend of scientific development and progress continued in the Islamic world with the great efforts of many dedicated Muslims, such as Muhammad Ibn Zakariyya AI-Razi (865-925 CE), described as the most creative genius of medieval medicine, whose masterpiece *al-Judari wal-Hasba (Small Pox and Measles)* was considered the first of its kind; Hunayn Ibn Ishaq (809-873 CE), who specialised in general medicine, dentistry and ophthalmology; Ibn AI-Bayad Ibn Ahmad, who made significant contributions in the area of pharmacology and therapeutics; Ali Ibn Isah (1000 CE), one of the most notable ophthalmologists, whose classical work, *Memorial of Ophthalmology* was the most widely used reference textbook among ophthalmologists for more than five

---

180. Namely; Abubakar, Umar, Usman and Ali (RA).

centuries; Ibn Rushd (1126-1198 CE), whose major encyclopaedic medical work, *Al-Kulliyat fil-Tibb (Generalities of Medicine)*, gave valuable guidance on ophthalmology and immunity, and was known to the West as Averoes; and the master physician, Abu Ali AI-Husayn Ibn Sina (980 - 1037 CE), who authored *AI-Qanunfi al-Iibb (The Canon of Medicine)* translated into many languages in many European medical schools, earning him the title, "Prince of Physicians."

The *Canon of Medicine* contained about two hundred and twenty-three (223) chapters devoted to many branches of medicine, ranging from surgery, therapeutics, paediatrics, orthopaedics, gynaecology, community health and pharmacology among others.

Apart from these eminent Muslim medical scientists, there are other erudite Muslim scholars who unsheathed their pens to elucidate the guidance of the Qur' an and Sunnah on medicine. Among them are Ali Ibn AI-Nafis (1210-1288 CE), who wrote *Sharh Tashrih al-Qanun (Commentary On the Analysis of the Canon of Avicenna);* Ibn Abi Usaybi'a (1203-1270 CE), *Uyun al-Anba'i fi Tabaqat al-Atibba (Sources of Information on the Classes of Physicians);* Imam Al-Bukhari (810-879 AD), who dedicated two chapters on medicine in his *Sahih* and Imam Malik (d. 795 AD), a chapter on Prophetic guidance on medicine in his *Muwatta.* Relatively, many independent works were contributed by Muslim scholars on *Tibbi Nabawi* (Prophetic Medicine), basing their contributions on the Sunnah of the Prophet (SAW) and his *Sahaba.* Such works, for example, include *Kitabul Shifa' a (Book of Healing)* of Imam Ghazzali; the *Tibbi Nabawi* of Imam Abu Nu'aim Al-Asfahani (d. 1038 CE); Imam Ibn Qayyim Al-Jawziyya (1292-1350 CE); Imam Jalaluddin As-Suyuti (b. 848 AH/I445 CE) among others.

Following the phase of rapid acquisition and dissemination of medical science by Muslim scholars, a generation of Muslim leaders emerged who were dedicated and committed to this Islamic spirit of pursuit of knowledge as a sacred duty. Among them, mention must be made of the Abbasid Caliph, Ma'moun (d. 813 CE), who founded *Dar al-Hikma* (The Hospice of Medical Treatment) in Baghdad, which included a medical college headed by a Muslim physician. Thereafter, *Al-Nuri* Hospital in Damascus, Syria and the *Mansuri* Hospital in Cairo, Egypt, were established. These hospitals and colleges established the basis of medical practice at the time and became the fountain head of the acquisition of medical knowledge for almost three centuries. In fact, it is said that, at one time, Baghdad had about sixty (60) hospitals, while Cordoba had more than fifty (50). In addition to that, there were small libraries and private collections each boasting of no less than 100,000 books.[181]

In the late centuries, the contribution of Sokoto caliphate scholars deserve to be mentioned. It is said that, the triumvirate of Sheikh Usman bn Fodio, his brother, Sheikh Abdullahi bn Fodio and his son, Sultan Muhammad Bello, wrote about a dozen books on various aspects of medicine such as *Masalihal Insani, Ujalatul Rakibi Fi Tibbis-Sa'ibi, At-Tibbul-Hayyin fi-Aujalaini, At-Tibbul-Nabawi, Alkaulul Sana, Adwiyatul Basur,* and so on. Sheikh Muhammad Tukur and Sheikh Umar bn Muhammad Bukhari (the eldest son of Sheikh bn Fodio) also wrote about five (5) books on general medicine, and Nana Asma'u, his daughter, also wrote and translated valuable works on medicinal remedies.[182]

The influence of all these Muslim scientists on the Eastern and Western European scientists and scholars who are today

---

181. *See* Al-akkili's translation of *Tibbi Nabawi* of Imam Ibn Qayyim.
182. There are many other similar works by Muslim, but the above suffice, since our intention is not merely to glorify past achievement or to lament over a pathetic loss, but to appreciate the potential that are inherent within us which need to be developed for good, instead of the pursuit of the frivolous and transient.

regarded as great contributors on different aspects of general science (medicine inclusive) is obvious. Yet, either by acts of omission or commission, the West deliberately made every effort to erase these historical facts. H.G.Farmer in his book, *Historical Fact in the Arabian Musical Influence,* wrote:

> *One of the most deplorable things in history is the systematic way in which European writers have contrived to put out of sight the scientific obligations of the Muslims.*

Nonetheless some Western scientists and orientalists have now come to realise the debt which Europe owe to the Muslims for their scientific and technological development. However, the fact still remains that Muslims have lost to the West their glory and intellectual heritage in science and technology. The following quotations are reminiscent of that past glory. Professor E.A. Badoe and his colleagues, while outlining the developmental milestones of medicine, in *The Principles and Practice of Surgery in the Tropics,* wrote:

> *With the fall of the Roman Empire and the rise and spread of CHRISTIANITY, the lamp whose rays were gradually shedding light on the mysteries of man and science was extinguished and medicine and surgery were plunged in almost complete darkness for a millennium. In the heyday of ISLAM from the 8th to 13th century, Arabic authors produced Arabic versions of Greek texts and a few of their own. During the medieval awakening these Arabic*

textbooks for a time were the fountain of medical knowledge.[183]

It is also recorded by A.H. Mayer in *History of Embryology* that:

> *From the time of Gwen (circa 200 AD) until the 16th century, no major advances in our knowledge of embryology were recorded in the literature of Western science. In point of fact, were it not for the Muslim writers many of the Greek works would have been lost to us.*

Robert Briffalut in his well known book, *The Making of Humanity,* wrote:

> *Science was the most important contribution of Arab civilisation to the modern world. Although there is not a particular aspect of the European blossoming whose origin cannot be ascribed to the influence of Islamic culture, these influences are found most clearly and most significantly in that capacity which has furnished the modern world with its enduring and distinctive power: namely, the natural sciences and the spirit of scientific inquiry.*

He then goes on to say:

> *Our science owes to that of the Arabs not amazing discoveries or original theories but something much more important - its existence.*

Professor Dreyber in his book, *The Struggle Between Religion and Science,* wrote:

---

183.   *See Principles and practice of Surgery in the Tropics* by Badoe *et al,* 2nd ed. pp.

We will be amazed to see in the writings of the Muslims, scientific theories which we thought to be the product of our age.

A.M.L. Stoddard on page 13 of *The New World of Islam,* wrote:

... the ancient cultures of Greece, Rome and Persia were revitalized by the Arab genius and the Islamic spirit. For the first three centuries of its existence (Circ. A.D. 650-1000) the realm of Islam was the most civilised and progressive portion of the world. Studded with splendid cities, gracious mosques and quiet universities, the Muslim World offered a striking contrast to the Christian West, then sunk in the night of the Dark Ages. [184]

Victor Robinson on page 164 of his book, *The Story of Medicine,* wrote as follows:

Europe was darkened at sunset, Cordova[185] *shone with public lamps; Europe lay in mud, Cordova's streets were paved; Europe's nobility could not sign its name, Cordova's children went to school; Europe's monks could not read the baptismal service, Cordova's teachers created a library of Alexandrian dimensions.*[186]

H.G. Weels in his *book, The Outline of History,* says:

---

184. *The New World of Islam,* London, 1932, pp 13.
185. The Capital of Spain during the Muslims' reign.
186. The Muslim Universities of Al- Azhar, in Egypt, and Cordoba in Spain, were established in the 10th century, about ttree hundred (300) years before the establishment of the Universities of Paris

... From a new angle and with a fresh vigour, the Arabs[187] took up that systematic development of positive knowledge which the Greeks had begun and relinquished. Through the Arabs it was and not by the Latin route that the modern world received that gift of light and power.

M.D. Anderson in his book, *Through The Microscope*, also noted the contributions of the Muslims in the field of Microbiology and Ophthalmology. He wrote:

After the decline of the Graeco-Roman civilization some progress was recorded in the study both of the eye and of glass lenses among the learned men of the Arab Empire.

Iswariah and Guruswani on page 4 of their book, *Pharmacology and Pharmaco-therapeutics*, wrote:

Physicians like Avicenna (1100 AD) exerted considerable influence in the medical world in the early Christian era. Even now we have relics of Arab influence in therapeutics in various names like alcohol, alkali, tartar, etc. The art of distillation is a legacy from the Arabs. The conquest of Spain by the Moors extended medical knowledge over the whole of the northern coastline of Africa and southern Europe. Mediaeval medicine was thus born and

187. It should be noted that Western writers use the terms Muslims or Arabs synonymously. This deliberate error should be disregarded because the scope of Islam is far wider than restricting it to the Arabs. Islam, though originated from Arabia, is a universal regardless of race, tribe, nation or any human barrier.

universities began to function and teach medicine.

George Sarton on page 17 of his book, *Introduction to the History of Science*, wrote:

In Islam, religion and science do not go their separate ways. In fact the former provided one of the main incentives for the latter. Muslim history thus furnishes no instance of the persecution of the scientists.

Again, Hartwig Hirschfield in his book, *Qur'an: The Fountain Head of the Sciences*, wrote:

We must not be surprised to find the Qur'an the fountain head of the sciences. Every subject connected with heaven or earth, human life, are occasionally touched. In this way the Qur' an was responsible for the development of all the branches of science in the Muslim world. This again not only affected the Arabs, but also induced Jewish philosophers to treat metaphysical and religious questions after Arab methods. In the same manner, the Qur'an gave an impetus to medical studies and recommended the contemplation and study of nature in general.

Thus, it is to the Muslim scientists that Europe has been in a great measure indebted for its extrication from the darkness of the middle ages. The realisation of the fact that the Muslims have for about a thousand years leave an indelible landmark in the progress of man in all aspects of life, should serve as an encouragement upon the present generation of Muslims to reclaim their lost glory and to strive to reach that level of higher humanity, which it, once attained in the course of its history. The Qur'an has enjoined us not to over-emphasise upon the past but to draw lessons from it.

> *That was a people that have passed away. They shall reap the fruit of what they did and you of what you do and you shall not be asked about what they did (Q2: 134).*

Muslims need to be reminded that the glory and dignity occupied by early Muslims were not attained by extraordinary means and unrepeatable miracles, but by means of a path corresponding to their own nature, efforts and human exertion and within the boundaries of human capacities. Yes, what happened once can happen again!

> *Do they not travel through the land, so that their hearts and minds may thus learn wisdom and their ears may thus learn to hear? (Q22:46).*

Historical occurrences repeat themselves and resemble each other because they are governed by consistent laws which set them in motion and adjust them. This is why people say, "History repeats itself." Dr Yusuf Al-Qaradawi in his book, *Islamic Awakening between Rejection and Extremism,* commented on the relevance of analysing historical fact:

A history of a nation, with all its positive and negative aspects, its victories and defeats, is a rich mine upon which that nation draws (lessons) in order to reconstruct and redirect its present. A nation that neglects its history is like a person who has lost his memory. This is why the Qur'an has given a special attention to the impact of the historical perspective and the wisdom that can be drawn from it.

Thus, victory is based on human efforts and exertion within the boundaries of human nature. The natural laws of Allah and His ways of granting victories to men are the same in all cases, and apply to all people irrespective of their religion, region or race. This is what the Qur'an meant by "man has nothing but what he strives for." [188] This is the truth God wished to teach the Muslims, and it is the same truth which He taught the early Muslim community at the battle of Uhud when it failed to represent the true nature of the faith in its self, and neglected the Prophet's advice at certain stages in the battle.[189] By neglecting or forgetting the primary truth, imaging that victory was a consequence of their being Muslims; Allah clearly pointed out this as an error and misunderstanding of Islam.

> *When a disaster befall you..., you exclaimed: 'Whose fault was that?' Say to them: "It was your own fault. Allah has power over all things"* (Q3: 165).

And so:

> *Whatever misfortune happens to you, is because of the things your hands have wrought (Q42:30).*

---

188. Qur'an 53:39
189. The Muslim community learnt this truth, albeit a hard and bitter lesson, not by words of reproach but through blood and suffering.

The consistency of Allah's Sunnah is therefore the common factor for all. It is in His own wisdom that He ordered nature into unchangeable laws and mechanisms.-

The nature made by Allah in which He has made men; there is no altering in Allah's creation (Q30:30).

And His saying:

But no change will you find in Allah's way (of dealing) (Q35:43).

Thus, Islam teaches that Muslims are not to be concerned only with Islamic history, but with the whole history of humanity, that of Muslims and non-Muslims, ever since the beginning of creation. Wisdom and lessons are not drawn from the history of believers alone, but from both the righteous and the profligate, because Allah's natural laws (of victory, and defeat, failure and success) operate upon both parties as stated earlier based on certain natural laws and fulfilment of certain conditions.

Many were the examples that have passed away before you; travel through the earth, and see what is the end of those who rejected truth (Q3:137).

And:

We have already sent down to you ... an illustration from the (story of) people who passed away before you, and an admonition for those who fear (Allah) (Q24:34).

It is true that humanity has today scored great triumphs, thanks to science, in the field of medicine and the physical cure of diseases. It has discovered new drugs and the means of diagnosis and treatment, and is now making a forward leap into the unbelievable era of genetic engineering and manipulation. But all these and more to come will not solve the problem of mankind, nor its blatant fight against diseases both known and unknown. This is because science without religion is a hallow tunnel incapable of taking man to the desired path of purity and prosperity. On the other hand, it is' also true that science from the beginning of the present century, has begun to lead great scientists back towards God. In spite of this spiritual reawakening and development, the dazzlement still remains that while previous generations were condemned for their ignorance and adoration of it, this generation would be judged for its knowledge and misappropriation of it.

There is no doubt that, more than ever before, humanity today is in need of the divine guidance of holy scriptures on all matters, particularly those related to science and technology. The extraordinary scientific achievements in particular and the challenges of the modern age have made the profligate to assume that science is superior to religion, or that man is not in need of God or His guidance for his survival and prosperity in this world. But Islam as a comprehensive way of life considers it a false claim that religion is not an essential requirement of this present age. The preference of science to the divine guidance is a denial of Allah as the Creator, and His rejection as the source of all knowledge.

Say! Do you know better than Allah? (Q2:140).

Against this background and historical fact, we know that Islam is not in conflict with science or any knowledge that is of benefit to man, except when such knowledge rejects Allah and the divine truth.

> Say: "Who has forbidden the beautiful gifts of Allah which He has produced for His servants, and the things clean and pure which He has provided for sustenance?" (Q7:32).

Here it is worth noting that there are some scholars who hold the erroneous belief that in order to attain the realm of spiritual blessings, one has to sacrifice the material things of this world and remain totally and holistically devoted to the hereafter. This concept is totally unacceptable. Moreover, Allah the Most High has refuted it in His book by commanding us thus:

> But seek, with that (wealth) which Allah has bestowed on you, the home of the hereafter, and forget not your portion of lawful enjoyment in this world; and do good as Allah has been good to you ... (Q28:77).

From this verse, it is now made clear that to be God-conscious does not mean to withdraw from the usual processes of life, nor to perform deeds which are utterly devoid of utilitarian value. The whole matter of religion from the Islamic point of view is to enhance the very quality of human life. Thus, Islam is the religion of rational and critical minds and the straightforward path chosen by Allah for the entire humanity. It is a religion of balance that enjoins man to seek for the goodness of this world and the hereafter concurrently. As a result, Islam neither approves of the pursuit of spiritually at the expense of material needs based on reality, nor of the tendency to purify the soul by neglecting the body. This is made very clear in the Qur'an:

Our Lord! Give us the good in this world and the good in the hereafter (Q2:201).

It is indeed very unfortunate that Muslims have not been able to mobilise and utilise the abundant human and material resources God has bestowed upon them for the guidance of humanity in all aspects of life. It is in such a situation of confusion and disunity, that the eternal guidance of the Qur'an is neither critically studied nor utilised for the progress of men. This is a very damaging and negative development, which still afflicts the Muslim Ummah.

Consequently, the progress of Muslims appears to be very slow or even stagnant in comparison to the quick strides of other nations. In spite of all these calamities, Muslims have good reasons to believe that the glorious Qur'an is the master book of all revelations and the standard for measuring all truths - scientific or otherwise. The future of Islam is the future of humanity, and if humanity has any future, which I believe it has, then there is a great and bright future in store for Islam - but not without the guidance of the Qur'an and Sunnah.

This day have I perfected your religion for you, completed My favour upon you and I have chosen for you Islam as your religion (Q5:3).

So if you differ in any matter among yourselves, refer it to Allah and His messenger for final determination (Q4:59).[190]

---

190. Meaning to consult the holy Qur'an and Sunnah of the prophet (SAW).

9.2 The Challenges of Modern Medicine to Muslims

From the foregoing, we have noticed the astonishing remarkable and unprecedented intellectual output in the various fields of medicine by the early Muslims. This is in accordance with the teachings and commandments of the Qur' an and Sunnah as a sacred duty to acquire and disseminate knowledge. One will then begin to wonder that in spite of the continuous appeal of the Qur' an, which we always read, and the practical demonstrations offered by the Sunnah, which we always adore, Muslims are still lagging behind in the areas of science and technology, particularly medicine. Dr Usman Bugaje in his Guest Speaker's address at the Annual Conference of the Islamic Medical Association, held at Usmanu Danfodiyo University, Sokoto, lamented over this pathetic situation:

From producers of knowledge, science and technology, we (Muslims) have today become consumers, poor ones at that, of knowledge, science and technology produced by a culture and civilisation that has no place, much less, role for the very Lord and Creator of man and the universe.[191]

How truthful! In this direction, Muslims should reflect on history and see whether we emulate our predecessors or not. Thus, in order to meet up with the challenges of modern medicine and the demands of the present world, Muslims must reflect upon the past, present and future and -recognise their responsibilities, limitations and potentialities. A firm faith in Allah and a sound knowledge are the fundamental requirements for combating this challenge:

191. Being part of Guest Speaker's address: "Some Contributions of Sokoto Caliphate Scholars to the Study Medicine," delivered at the Opening Ceremony of the Annual Conference of the Islam Medical Association, Usmanu Danfodiyo University, Sokoto, in 1995.

> *Obey Allah and His Messenger and fall into no disputes, lest you loose your heart and your power depart you (Q8:46).*

In Islam, faith in God, an ever-revealing source of knowledge and insight into countless fields of thought, is the cornerstone of the whole religious structure and success of man's life in this world and the next. Moreover, Islam does not recognise faith when it is attained without true knowledge based on clear proofs and evidence acquired by experience or experiment. In this connection it is safe to say, beyond doubt, that the Qur'an is the first religious authority to enjoin a zealous quest for knowledge through experience, experiment, meditation, observation and research. Islam awakens in man the faculty of reason, nourishes the spirit of inquisitiveness and exhorts him to use his intellect. It enjoins man to see things in the light of reality. The Qur'an enjoins man to pray:

> *O Lord! Increase me in knowledge (Q20: 114).*

It is amazing that in spite of the continuous appeal of the Qur'an and Sunnah to Muslims to seek for and utilise ~e virtues of knowledge, Muslims still remain backward in the areas of science and technology. In fact, for the past few centuries the Muslim world has lived in a very pathetic and deplorable state. From whatever perspective one chooses to view the Ummah, be it political, economic, educational or social, one can see that it is placed at the "lowest rung of the ladder of nations." Yet, a cursory glance at history reveals that it was the solid scientific attitude which Islam encompasses that gave the necessary thrust very early in Islamic history, which motivated Muslims to forge ahead in all academic spheres, and to produce scholarly works in all fields of human endeavour or disciplines such as medicine, philosophy, science and the social Sciences.

The underlying Islamic world view provided a conducive environment for the different disciplines to develop in a rapid and constructive way during the first few centuries of Islam. Crucial to this development in scientific knowledge was a thorough understanding of their missions as the vicegerents of Allah on earth. Equally important was the availability of the tools of *ijtihad* and their ability to extract from the Qur'an and Sunnah a solid methodology not only for deriving knowledge through experimentation and reasoning, but also for dealing with knowledge that had already been developed by other civilisations. This was the period when Islam was comprehensively put into practice, when the Qur'an J1; self played a leading role in translating the ideas of Islam into reality, all in making this period of history an era which posterity could refer to and strive to emulate.

However, with time, the Muslim Ummah began to decline politically and economically, and the conducive environment for learning and research ceases to continue. This paves the way for the intellectual decline of the Muslim Ummah, and the Muslim world came to a standstill. The void created allowed the Western world to forge ahead and take over the position of the Muslims in leading the rest of the world in different spheres of knowledge and development. There is no doubt that the imposition of western civilisation (in all aspects) on the Muslim world by means of colonisation has had serious destructive consequences on Muslims. It is however clear that the most harmful and destructive aspects of it all is the educational or intellectual aspect because it ensures the perpetuation of political, economic and cultural subjugation of the Muslim world to the West.

Another crucial factor in this intellectual decline and the erosion of the rich Muslim heritage is the closure of the door of *Ijtihad* and the adoption of full-scale *Taqlid* by some scholars. Then there arose another factor which came from the sincere but ignorant Muslim who thinks that the best way to defend religion is by rejecting all the sciences. This led to the misconception on the part of the scientists that Islam has ignorance and the denial of scientific proofs as its basis. This attitude encourages dissatisfaction with religion among the scientists, and the rejection of its divine teachings.

On the other hand, there is the role and attitude of the Muslim modernists (apologetics of the West) who advocate total adoption of and adaptation to Western thoughts and ideas, and the forceful interpretation of Islamic texts to conform to them. This is actually a manifestation of intellectual apathy and psychological defeat that do more harm to Islam than good. More importantly, the moral decadence of some Muslim rulers and leaders who neglected Islamic teachings and become fully devoted a to materialism and the pursuit of worldly desires, without doubt, constitutes a great stumbling block to the progress of Islam and the Muslim Ummah.

> *There is certainly a lesson in their story for people who have understanding. It is not a tale invented, but a confirmation of what went before it (Q12:111).*

Thus, it is not surprising that the Muslims of today are far behind the developed countries of Europe and America in science and technology, in spite of the constant and repeated commandments in the Qur'an anti Sunnah that Muslims should earnestly seek for knowledge. There is abundant evidence even in Western literature (as presented earlier) that the West received the stimulus for scientific research from the Muslims, but the Muslims of latter generations failed to develop, perfect and convert it to greater invention as the Europeans did in the course of their history. Consequently, the Muslims became idle spectators, lazy and worldly and ultimately were overwhelmed and enslaved by the rising powers of Europe and America. This could not have been possible but for the fact that Muslims disregarded the teachings of Islam, having forgotten their position of vicegerency on earth, and failed to fulfil the injunctions of Allah and His Messenger (SAW):

> *Verily never will Allah change the condition of a people until they change what is in themselves (Q13:11).*

And:

> *Because Allah will never change the grace which He has bestowed on a people until they change what is in their own souls (Q8:53).*

The Prophet (SAW) also said:

> *He who practices what he knows Allah will cause him to inherit knowledge of what he did not know.*

Therefore, the only way forward for Muslims is to capture the essence of knowledge in its proper Islamic axis - for the Ummah to regain her lost glory. To attain the leadership of mankind, Muslims must have something to offer humanity a way of life which on the one hand conserves and develops the benefits of modern science and technology, and on the other, fulfils the basic human spiritual needs in the same level of excellence as technology has fulfilled in the sphere of material comfort. The Prophet had earlier said:

> *Knowledge is the lost property of the believer he should take it wherever he finds it.*[192]

When Islam demands faith in Allah on the basis of knowledge and research, it leaves wide open all the fields of thought before the intellect to penetrate as far as it can reach; lays down no restriction and urges man to resort to all methods of knowledge, be they purely rational or experimental. The Qur'an singles out the Muslim Ummah as the best community in this regard for enjoining what is good and forbidding evil.

> *You are the best community ever brought for mankind; you enjoin **al-ma arufand forbid al-munkar** (Q3:110).*

> We have made of you an Ummah justly balanced that you might be witnesses over the nations (Q2:143).

The Qur'an further states:

> *He hath chosen you and hath not laid upon you in religion any hardship. He has named you Muslims of old time and in this (scripture) that the messenger may be a witness for you, and that you be witnesses for mankind (Q22:78).*

---

192.   Reported from Abu Hurairah in Sahih Bukhari and Tirmidhi.

In order to fulfil the obligations of this "best and balanced community" and be witnesses over all nations, Muslims must aspire for the best in all respects. Today science and technology have become so crucial to the development of any society that the Muslim Ummah has no option but to fully engross itself in their pursuits, and lead other nations in this respect.

Then do you remember Me; I will remember you. Be grateful to Me and reject not faith (Q2: 152).

And strive in His cause as you ought to strive (with sincerity and under discipline) He has chosen you (as Muslims) and has imposed no difficulties on you in religion (Q22:78).

And:

Go you forth and strive and struggle with your goods and persons. That is best for you if you (but knew) (Q9:41).

9.3 The Principles and Approaches of "Islamic Medicine"

In Islam, Allah as the Creator, is the ultimate source of all knowledge and that man, by the nature bestowed on him by Allah, is only capable of acquiring and comprehending a limited portion of this knowledge. Hence, science as part of God-given knowledge to man will never be able to explain everything, neither will it always have the right answers. Up to date, in spite of the advanced level of medicine, there are so many diseases and disorders whose aetiology (causes) and pathogenesis (course) are still unknown and unexplained. For instance, in pharmacology (the study of drugs and their effects) there are many instances in which the knowledge of how some drugs act to effect a cure remain unknown or scientifically unexplainable. Therefore, medicine, like all other branches of knowledge in Islam, must be based on the principle of *Tawheed* (the Unity of God). This principle allows us to view science as a means of exploring the intricate design and order that our Creator, the best of all designers, has given to His creatures.

> We have indeed created man in the best of moulds (constitution) (Q95:4).

Behind this intricate design there must be a purpose, which becomes all the more evident as we go deeper into the study of medical science as well as other branches of knowledge. Imam Al-Ghazzali observed that, "Certainly no one can study anatomy and the wonderful mechanisms of living things without being obliged to confess to the profound wisdom of Him who has formed the bodies of animals, and especially of man," Al-Farabi also said, "Anybody who studies anatomy, his faith in the existence of Allah will increase."

Thus, true knowledge in Islam and medicine inspires in him, who is initiated in it, more fear and reverence, and raises a barrier of defence between him and sin. "A true Muslim seeks the truth of his profession," according to Imam Al-Ohazzali, "not by systematic reasoning and accumulation of proofs, but by the flash of light which God directs into his soul." This is the light and guidance which illuminate the threshold of all knowledge (medical science inclusive).

> And Allah guides whom He wills to a way straight (Q24:46).

It is He (Allah) who created me and it is He who guides me. And when I am sick, it is He who cures me (Q26:78 and 80).

And:

If Allah helps you, none can overcome you and if He forsakes you, who is there, after that, that can help you? In Allah, then let the believers put their trust (Q3: 160).

An Islamic oriented medical science must also recognise Allah as the cause and effect of all the rules governing the universe. The principle of causality and aetiology, which lies at the root of all scientific research, must not becloud this fact and reality, for there is nothing that happens without His permission.

Not an atom's weight in heaven or earth can escape His knowledge (Q10:61).

And:

Every misfortune that befalls the earth or your own person is ordained in a clear record, before We bring it into existence (Q57:12).

And:

He is the First and the Last, the Visible and the Unseen. He has knowledge of all things (Q57:3).

Aisha (RA) narrated in Sahih Bukhari that wherever Allah's Apostle (SAW) paid a visit to a patient, or a patient was brought to him, he used to invoke Allah, saying, "Take away the disease, O the Lord of the people; cure him as You are the One who cures. There is no cure but Yours, a cure that leaves no disease." It is reported by Abdullahi bn Umar in Sahih Muslim that Ummu Habiba (RA), the wife of the Prophet, prayed to Allah for longevity, on account of which the Prophet responded:

> *Verily you have asked Allah about the duration of life already set and the steps which you would take and the sustenance the share of which is fixed. Nothing would be taken, deferred or delayed beyond that which is ordained.*

On the other hand, Islam as a religion of balance and moderation encourages Muslims to strive and dominate the earth and utilise its resources and subdue their enemies both the seen and unseen or invisible creatures (which include the world of pathogens or disease causing micro-organisms). The Qur'an states:

> *Did you not see that Allah has made subservient to you all that is on the earth? (Q22:65).*

Another basic principle of Islamic teaching is the unity of knowledge, which in essence means Allah is the source of all knowledge. Thus, there is nothing like "Western knowledge" or secular knowledge as opposed to religious knowledge. Professor Jibril Aminu in his Guest Speaker's address during an International Seminar on "Islam and the Development of Science and Technology," attempts to make this clarification. He tells us:

> *It may have been observed that one has tried not to use the phrase 'Islamic Science and*

Technology' or anything with a similar connotation. This is because, in truth, there is no such thing, and there is no Islamic source that we are aware of that subscribes to such concept. Similarly, there is nothing like Christian or Western Science and Technology. Science is the same the world over, and has been so from the beginning of time because, it is the study and observation of fundamental truths. Technology, which could otherwise be termed human resourcefulness, is exactly the same in this respect. Science, after all, simply means knowledge. Science and technology, being universal, are truly world intellectual property belonging to everyone.[193]

Concerning this unified concept of knowledge (in term of its source) the Qur'an states:

He (Allah) taught man what he knows not (Q95:5).

And:

He has created man. He has taught him an intelligent speech (Q55:34).

What is meant to be put across here is that Allah has sent down knowledge, and He blessed man with the intellect and power of reasoning. If man uses this intelligence given to him appropriately he can explore and exploit the treasures of knowledge. Empirical knowledge could therefore be explored and acquired by man through experience. As for revealed knowledge, man can never attain it except by revelation from the Most High.

...It is only a little knowledge that is communicated to you (o mankind) Q17:85.

In spite of the common source for all kinds of knowledge, Muslim scholars have classified knowledge into varied groups based on its diversity and utilisation or application.[194] According to Imam AI-Ghazzali (450 A.H), there are two types of know ledge; religious and secular, and Islam enjoins and encourages acquiring both types of knowledge. That Islam places obligation for the acquisition of both, one on an individual basis (that is *Fard Ainih)* and the other on a collective basis (that is *fard Kifayat).*

Al-Alwani[195] alluded to this categorisation of knowledge, saying that the two are complementary to each other. There are no contradictions between the two, and each helps in the understanding of the other. He maintains that from the verses which command us to read:

---

194. This is not a contradiction of our earlier view of a unified concept of knowledge. In essence, the unity of knowledge is in terms of its source of knowledge come from Allah. However, in terms of its diversification and utilization, knowledge can be classified.
195. Prof. Taha Jabir Al-Alwani is an erudite scholar and author of many valuable works on the Islamisation of knowledge. He is the president of the international Institute of Islamic Though (IIIT), USA.

...It may be deduced that humanity has been commanded to undertake two different kinds of readings and to understand its situation in the universe through understanding of how the two complement one another. The first reading is the book of Allah's revelation (the Qur'an), in which all matters of religious significance are explained, and the second is the book of the creation (the natural universe). To undertake a reading of either without reference to the other will neither benefit humanity, nor lead it to the sort of comprehensive knowledge necessary for the building and the maintenance of civilised society, or to knowledge worthy of preservation and further development or exchange.

Sayyid Abul A'la Maududi in his book, *Towards Understanding Islam*, enlightened us further:

Islam regards knowledge and science as the common heritage of mankind, and the Muslims have the perfect liberty to learn them and their practical uses from whatever quarter they can.

From the above, it would be seen that Islam really views knowledge as a universal phenomenon. In other words, knowledge in its entirety and essence is a universal human heritage and no race, tribe, nations or colour has the monopoly of knowledge. So all human races, tribes or nations could excel in terms of exploring, acquiring, transforming and developing knowledge. It is simply a matter of historical evolution that one race or community dominates others in terms of educational development. In the same vein it is a matter of adventurism, hard work and seriousness with life.

This is a historical fact which could be proven by making reference to the memories of Egyptian, Persian, Greek, Roman and Islamic civilisations.

It is therefore made clear that the realisation of some of the divine gifts has been left to human exertions. Failure to understand this simple truth leads to a whole series of questions: Is Islam not revealed by God? Is God not omnipotent? Why then does Islam operate only within the boundaries of restricted human abilities? 'Why should the result of its operation be affected by human weakness? Why is it not always triumphant or its followers not always on the lead? Why should its course on certain occasion be overcome by material realities? Why do those in the wrong sometimes triumph over the righteous? All these questions arise in the first place from misunderstanding the nature of Islam and its mode of operation.

Islam teaches that man is not a mere puppet in the mighty hand of nature. God in His infinite wisdom and mercy has conferred upon man a limited autonomy, according to which he is free to do or not to do certain things. The concept of predestination *(Qadr)* in Islam, therefore, does not in any way mean the helpless abandonment of oneself to otherwise unwelcome fate. It rather means co-operation with God, studying His will and bringing oneself into unison with His planning and will. This unity between human efforts and destiny, is implied in Allah's statement:

> *Allah does not change the condition of a people until they change it themselves (Q8:53).*
> *And that each man shall be judged by his own labours (Q53:39).*

It is therefore mandatory for the Muslims to shake off, if any, despondency and despair, and unfold their inherent potentialities in the vast fields of human endeavour. That in the world today the secular nations of the East and West are more advanced scientifically and technologically than the Muslim nations is but a manifestation of the natural law of Allah and His impartial grace and blessings - a revolving opportunity which He offers to peoples and communities at different stages of the world's history.

> *The bounties of thy Lord are never withheld from anyone (Q17:20).*

> *For every nation a space of time is fixed, when their hour comes not for one moment shall they hold it back, nor can they go before it (Q7:34).*

We must content ourselves with the world's history and reflect on how the high tide of Islam passed away, and how other nations again held the reins of power through the tools of science and technology. It is the duty of the Muslim nations to tell the world about Islam; that universal phenomenon, which for the first time abolished all man-made barriers and united mankind, promoted global peace and prosperity and remained for more than a thousand years a source of inspiration and encouragement. It opened up vast fields of human activity from which other societies sought help. History bears witness to that. That path, that guidance and that struggle is alive even if it had retreated from its position of dominance in the world. Yes, Muslims have in the Qur'an and Sunnah the greatest potentialities capable of re-writing the course of history.

> *Seek help from Allah and be patient, the earth belongs to Allah, He gives to those of His servants whom He chooses (Q7:128).*

The conclusion arrived at in this respect is that, it is the primary duty of every Muslim at individual or community or even global level to appreciate the facts of human history, understand their line of development on the one hand, and how to confront and influence it, on the other hand. As a prerequisite to that understanding, it must also be appreciated that the unique forward leap of Islam was not the result of an unrepeatable miracle, rather it was the fruit of human exertion made by the first Muslim community. Such a lofty peak can be achieved whenever a similar exertion is made. This unique path of Islam at all times is still capable of producing such ideal men and society, as long as serious efforts are made irrespective of all opposing factors and obstacles. This environment is suitable to the rise of such a generation provided the Qur' an and Sunnah are appropriately and properly utilised. Yes, by Allah, what happened once can happen again.

And fulfil your covenant with Me, and I shall fulfil My covenant with you (Q2:240).

9.4 The Islamisation of the Medical Sciences

Although it is said earlier that knowledge is universal, it is however noteworthy to affirm that despite its universality, it bears a cultural stamp. Every human community has its own exclusive cultural values and peculiar civilisational orientation. Subsequently, societies and communities differ in their respective approach and views about knowledge and what it stands for. On the basis of its cultural values and aspirations, a community delineates its aims and objectives and methods of acquiring knowledge as well as the structure and contents of its educational system. It is well known that in order to determine the degree of the consonance of Western education to the Islamic value system, even a superficial analysis will show that it depends on human reasoning and intellect alone as the source of knowledge. It mocks at the idea of a supreme Being who is the Creator and Controller of the universe.[196]

Thus, a scientific world view cannot be the foundation for a human ideology. This is because the value of scientific knowledge is primarily practical, in that it enables man to dominate nature, but it is unable to show man a direction in life that harmonises matter and spirit. Today, the spiritual poverty of man is advancing at a rate commensurate with his scientific and technological wealth. As man progressed in industry and science, he regressed in ethics and spirituality, to such a degree that he lacked the moral capacity to make a proper use of his newly acquired knowledge. Hence, scientific knowledge infused with Western civilisation, is in itself indifferent to values and ethics and therefore one cannot determine the duties of a responsible human being by referring to science alone. However far science advances, it cannot see more than one step ahead of itself because its educational foundation is materialism and the denial of God. Of all systems and beliefs, it is only the Islamic world view that does not attempt to confine man to the material or spiritual aspects of his existence to the detriment of the other.

This makes it necessary for Muslims to attempt to reorient and recast knowledge to conform to the Islamic belief system and world view.[197] So that medical sciences (as well as the other branches of science) are channelled to go after knowledge that will be beneficial to humanity. This was the noble tradition that our early Muslim doctors and scientists

---

196. See "The Islamic Vision of Knowledge – Its Implication and Signi-fication to the Islamisation of Knowledge Programme." A Paper Presented at a Seminar on Isamisation of Knowledge, Bayero University, Kano, Nigeria.
197. See "Isamisation of the Natural sciences – Myth or Reality." A Paper Presented at a Seminar on Islamisation of Knowledge at Bayero University, Kano, Nigeria.

strictly adhered to in the past. It was in keeping with this principle that Al-Razi, the great Muslim scientist, firmly refused to prepare poisons even though he had the ability to do so.

Another challenge is related to a certain aspect of the advances of modern medicine which raised many serious problems. What should we do at a time when surrogate motherhood, organ transplantation, milk banking, artificial insemination, blood transfusion, plastic surgery, sex, selection or determination and frightening advances in genetic engineering, etc are revolutionising the principles and practice of medicine? Genetic engineering and cloning, for example, have the prospect of making it possible to "shop for a baby in the same way we shop for the latest design in the cloth industry," and to specifically choose the sex of the baby needed for conception, and to modify the baby's characteristics and susceptibility to certain diseases. Do we have the intellectual capacity to address or combat these challenges?

Thus, an important approach to take up the challenges posed by medicine to present day Muslims bothers on adventurism, hardwork and seriousness. Given the wide gap and the fundamental differences which exists between the Islamic and secular approaches to knowledge, it is right to say a herculean task lay ahead for the Muslims, provided we are intent on reclaiming (not merely glorifying) our lost treasure. Since secularism has been the basic foundation upon which Western philosophy and the methodology of knowledge are built, religion has obviously and systematically been downplayed and relegated to the background. This being a consequence of the great controversy between men of science and the church, the victory of the former over the latter has made the Western world to believe that religion and all it stands for was reactionary, retrogressive, backward and superstitious, and that it has exhausted all its usefulness and must therefore surrender to science.

This trend came to be the major characteristic of the Western approach to knowledge and its relationship with religion. But it has been demonstrated in the preceding passages, the Islamic vision of knowledge, the intellectual and the unprecedented inputs of the Muslim scientists and doctors towards the development of science and scientific attitude and enquiry. What this implies is that, since Muslims have had such a sublime, independent, dynamic and fundamental system of knowledge they must try to develop, process and transform it into a higher level for the benefit of the Ummah, and its presentation to the global community.

> Say: *Truly, my prayer and my service of sacrifice, my life and my death, are (all) for Allah, the Cherisher of the worlds (Q6:162).*

> *The baptism of Allah - and who can baptise better than Allah? It is He, whom we worship (Q2: 138).*

This is the basis for the Islamisation of knowledge.

CHAPTER TEN

Conclusion

It is seen that collectively the Qur' an and Sunnah show through many methods, means and manner, how the health of humanity can be improved. This further shows that the Glorious Qur'an is a source of scientific information meant to be utili sed for the progress of man. This unique characteristic of the Qur' an calls for thought and reflection, and also casts a light on its divine origin.

How is it possible that the teachings of an unlettered Arab, about 1400 years ago, should be in agreement with modern scientific findings, particularly on health? The Prophet could not have known these facts in the 7th century, since most remarkable discoveries in the history of medicine were recorded only in the 20th century. Truly the Qur' an is a revelation from God:

This is the book which We have revealed unto you (Muhammad) in order that you might lead mankind out of the depths of darkness into light (Q14:1).

Muslim scholars stated that it was called "Al-Qur'an" from among the Books of God not because it gathered the fruit of other holy books, but because it gathered the fruits of all knowledge. Allah the Almighty has confirmed this when He described the Qur'an as:

a detailed exposition of all things (Q12: 111).

Surely Muhammad (SAW) is a messenger sent by Allah to all mankind. This fact is further proven by his practical demonstration of Allah's message to humanity in an excellent manner. In view of the knowledge in Muhammad's day, it is inconceivable that many of the scientific statements of the Qur'an could have any human author.

The recognition that Islamic ideology motivates humanity to pursue knowledge and investigate natural laws and phenomena in various scientific fields has been a great contribution to humanity. In the same manner Islam gave an impetus to medical studies which the Prophet (SAW) referred to as "the knowledge of the body," and recommended the contemplation and study of nature in general. This characteristic nature of Islam made it a unique system of life covering a whole spectrum of issues which range from specific articles of faith, moral teachings, rights and obligations, law and relations, science and the universe and a host of other private and social concerns. As a result of this, scholars, both Muslims and non-Muslims through the generations, have dedicated themselves wholeheartedly to the study of the Qur'an and Sunnah in the light of modern science. It is as an extension of these efforts that this book attempts to provide an insight into the Qur'anic passages and the traditions of the Prophet (Sunnah) related to the field of medicine. Thus, it is our hope that through this book the Qur'anic message and the practical demonstration of the

Sunnah of the Prophet (SAW), with regards to the practice and principles of medicine, have been conveyed. It is also shown that the backwardness of Muslims in medicine and other branches of knowledge is not the resultant effect of the deficiency of Islam as a religion, but of the Muslims' inability to utilise its guidance and consistent appeal for action.

The revival of Islamic teachings in the field of Medicine will restore for the Muslim heart its spirit that was lost after science had been detached from religion, and the whole Muslim Ummah has became an ymmah of consumption and importation of everything, including medicine. The Muslim physician finds no nourishment in his heart, and the patient in his hands turned into a collection of separate systems and organs instead of a human being of one entity, consisting of body and soul. Due to the absence of that comprehensive view, many physical diseases appeared while they are mere reflections of psychological disorders.

Allah has endowed the Muslim world with a huge wealth of medicinal plants which can provide cures for all diseases afflicting mankind. Some of these medicinal plants described by Ibn Sina, Al-Razi, Al-Biruni, and many others, have been studied and tested by previous medical scholars in several centres of learning. There is the need for the evaluation of these plants according to the 21st century scientific criteria and requirements. The initiative is now open to the Muslims of the world to assert themselves and see that the 21st century of the Christian era, or the 15th century of the Islamic, will show that our "forty years of wandering in the wilderness" has now ended, and we are now ready to join, and possibly lead the rest of the world in ushering a new era, the harbinger of material and spiritual prosperity for all mankind.

In order for Muslims to take up the challenges facing the Ummah in the sphere of modern medicine among other branches of science and technology development, we must, as a matter of priority, begin to put our own house in order, so that we not only survive in the midst of this new opportunity and its challenge, but also take over our leadership status. The problems of disunity, sectarian conflicts, instability, underdevelopment, hunger, disease, ignorance and general poverty that plague most of the Muslim world, and indeed most of the Third World, must be addressed. The Islamic world desperately needs to reorganise itself. Muslim countries and well-to-do individual Muslims and organisations must be more serious and committed towards promoting education and financing research and development. Seriousness is an ingredient without which any amount of investment in human and material resources will be useless.

Moreover, the relationship between the Muslim world and the West needs to be redefined in order to promote mutual and bilateral co-operation. The West need a fresh study of Islam divorced from the ideas of the Crusades. There has been much criticism of Islam over the years and even over the centuries. For long Islam and Muslims have suffered from an "image problem" because the West, which controls the global media, has chosen to deliberately misunderstand Islam. Western people must learn to understand the Muslims with whom they share the planet. Western idea about Islam have been crude, dismissive and prejudicial. Therefore, the old literature which has been published about Islam by Orientalists, who studied Islam with a mindset guided (or misguided) by morbid hatred and prejudice, needs to be re-written or at least revisited and made more objective and "scientific," so as to make the idea of "live and let live" meaningful.

The attitude of the West tends to confirm the belief of many Muslims that they were, and are still, reluctant to study Islam, except in their own mistaken textbooks. Anyone who insists on labelling Islam "medieval" and making it look inadequate for modern conditions is living in a mythical world of his own. If Europe and America prefer to continue thinking of Islam in the old fashion, repeating old cliches about four wives, a holy war (a misnomer for *Jihad*), an epileptic theory of the source of the Qur' an, and so on, the world will soon pass them by.

It is, therefore,· advisable to have a scientific and rational approach to Islam. Islam is quite easy to understand if it is taken on its own merit. Islam has penetrated into every nook and cranny of the globe and has contributed excellently well to every field of human learning. Islam, the fastest growing religion in the world, has inspired as many scholars, professors and scientists as mystics and poets. It is unarguably the basis for humanity's illustrious civilisation. The non-Muslim world must therefore endeavour to understand Islam properly. Islam should be seen as an all-embracing culture, and as a vast synthesising agent at work on the peoples it has touched and brought together in harmony. Islam should be viewed as a key, not as a barrier, to understanding science and technology.

Just as the rest of the world is being called upon to adjust to Islam and Muslims, it is equally necessary for Muslims to adjust to the changing environment, regain their self-confidence in order to deal effectively and constructively with the world around them. This implies that the Muslim world must relate with the rest of the world for its own sake. Insulation, isolation or dissociation is illogical, considering the fact that, today, there is hardly any society or country in the world which can totally be independent of others. Muslims would have to come to terms with Western society, their technological breakthrough and scientific progress because these were facts of life. We must see clearly with "open" eyes so as to make a clear distinction between what is evil in the West, and what is really a continuation of that quest for knowledge, of which Islam in the middle ages was the principal champion.

To reject knowledge, whatever its source, is to repudiate one of the principles enunciated by Islam. It is easy indeed to condemn modern science and technology in vague and abstract terms by associating every modern evil with them. But the equating of evil with science rests on false premises and prejudices which only an appeal to the concrete can expose. Yet, Muslims must take cognizance of "destructive sciences," whose consequences and effects are harmful to man and the environment, and are against the natural and moral laws of the universe. This has been the tradition of early Muslim scientists and scholars.

Therefore, the Muslim world, with such a brilliant past behind it and a bright future in sight, must proudly raise its banner among the greatest civilisations and cultures produced by man. We must fashion out a new direction - which on the one hand conserves and develops the benefits of modern science and technology, and on the other, fulfils the basic human spiritual needs in the same level of excellence, without losing our sense of identity.

Finally, it is hoped that both Muslims and non-Muslims will appreciate this remarkable feature of medicine in accordance with the Qur'an and Sunnah.

> *O Believers! Thrn to Allah together in repentance that you may prosper (Q24:31).*
>
> *Who listens to the distressed when he calls on Him and Who relieves his suffering and makes you inheritors of the earth (Q27:62).*

So lose not heart, nor fall into despair for you must gain mastery if you are true in faith (Q3:139).

Appendix

Authority of *Tibbi Nabawi* (Prophetic Medicine)

I deemed it necessary to comment on the authority or rather position of the prophetic medicine with regards to the issue of its practical application in the practice of contemporary medicine. Understanding this position is crucial in determining our approach to what came in the Islamic legislation about medicine in the light of current knowledge and the relation between faith and cure. It is noteworthy to state that the body of medical knowledge, the so-called "Islamic medicine" is in reality a blend of 3 distinct elements:

The Greek based tradition, which is the inheritance of preceding civilisations, particularly the Greek, preserved, developed and adopted by the Muslims.
Pre-Islamic cultural practices which refers to the folk or traditional medicine (customarily practised by the Arabs and associated tribes) prevalent before the rise of Islam, and continues thereafter. Lastly, the scriptural medicine which

is a referral to the medical guideline and pointers
drawn from the Qur' an and Sunnah addressing
such wide areas as curative, (use of honey),
preventive (cleanliness and hygiene), ethics (ban
on alcohol and sexual perversion), policy and
constitutional matters (leadership and account-
ability) and matters of spiritual dimensions
(prayers, invocation and supplication).

It is worth clarifying that some of our heritage books seem to address all these dichotomous ad distinct elements under the term "prophetic medicine." Yet, a representation of this body of knowledge under the blanket term "prophetic medicine" tends to more harm than good.

Firstly, to the uneducated masses, they are likely to accept everything uncritically as part of divine revelation whereas in reality it contains elements that are simply "quackery piously disguised." The rational disguise and its attributary to the Prophet make it all the more harmful. As to the scholars, particularly experts in medicine, this discovery will lead to the misconception that Islam has ignorance and denial of scientific proofs as its basis. This attitude becomes a seed for dissatisfaction with religion among the scientists, and the rejection of even divine teachings.

Here it is crucial to note that historically during their period of development, there seem to be an effort by Muslim scholars to supplement the flourishing Greek based medical practice and pre-Islamic Arab medical customs with something closely linked to divinely revealed knowledge. Thus, parallels with these practices whose influence began to decline by 7th and 8th centuries, prophetic medicine evolved to incorporate other materials that are not traceable to the Prophet himself or his closest companions. For instance, the humoral basis, which was a treasure of the Greek medical system, appeared in treatises specifically on prophetic medicine *(Tlbbi Nabawi),* such as that of Imam Ibn Qayyim AI-Jawziya and that of Imam Jalal AI-Din AI-Suyuti. There are also references to maladies being related to if not caused by black and yellow bile and phlegm. The narratives are replete with list of medicaments designed to alleviate such afflictions.

On its association with Arab traditional medical practice, mentioned must be made of the "evil eye," cupping and cauterisation, which in most narrations were strongly criticised by the Prophet himself. Related to this and without substantiation is the narration of the use of animal's (camel's) urine in treating the sick.

In addition to all these one may also find the infiltration of corrupt concepts into the pure prophetic medicine. For instance, there is evidence that magical properties has been conferred on such otherwise innocuous elements as the soil of the grave of the Prophet or his companions, the sighting of a saint by the afflicted, and so on.

The Shi'ite Muslim beliefs added another dimension into the prophetic medicine by its recognition of members of the family of the Prophet beginning with and through the line of Ali bn Abu Talib (the Prophet's cousin and son-in-law) as having been divinely designated to govern the Muslim community. Their statements, actions and prescriptions are therefore, regarded as divinely-inspired, and constitute both a commentary on and an extension of the revelation.

The belief even though not much different from the Sunni's regards for *ijtihad* through which pious scholars (regardless of their blood ties with the Prophet) exercise judgement in accordance with the spirit and letter of Islam, and such prescriptions are considered part of or subsumed in the Sunnah of the Prophet. In contrast to Shi'ite, wever, the divine inspiration is downplayed and the saints' infallibility denounced.

Quite clearly, the rise in prophetic medicine was related to or connected with the decline in Galenic medicine and the subsistence of arguments for its validity over the pre-Islamic Arab traditional medical practice. Thus, as the Galenic medicine declined, the third dichotomous tradition in Islamic medicine (the prophetic medicine) increasingly asserted itself. It is generally depicted as having arisen to counter the authority of the other medical traditions by positing that knowledge and certainty in medicine, as in religion and philosophy, could only be attained through, revelation. In spite of the obvious fact that prophetic medicine is not exclusively based on the Qur'an and the statements and actions of the Prophet, over-zealous scholars, in order to win more hearts and minds raise it to the status of a divine revelation.

This erroneous portrayal of prophetic medicine has become a basis for the misconception among the western scholars that "Islamic medicine" totally claims to be a divinely ordained prescription to which its adherents must be devotedly committed. As a result of prejudice and without a systematic comparative study of the Muslim holy scriptures, they portray "Islamic medicine" in relatively static, irrational and uncompromising terms. That this is not so is evident from authentic traditions which confirmed that the Prophet never claim absolute authority on (earthly) matters other than spiritual. This has been clearly demonstrated in his attempts at cross-breeding of date to improve yield as well as his caution against those who through misinformation take advantage of his judicial pronouncements. This attitude is visible in his encouragement for the utilisation of medical knowledge, skills and ideas (among other branches of knowledge) from both Muslims and non-Muslims. In fact, he has reputedly consulted and invited non-Muslim physicians to attend to him when sick.

A sincere seeker of truth will find out that while some of the actions and utterances of the Prophet on medical practice or its principles constitute the practical demonstrations of the Qur' anic guide, there are some that represent the practice, knowledge and norms of cultural setting of the day, which do not carry any divine indictment, but were naturally allowed or even encouraged to evolve in accordance with the time and space factor.

In this direction, I find it very relevant to refer to the views of renowned scholar, Professor Abdul Aziz Kamel, whose paper titled "Faith and Cure" appeared in the proceedings of the second international conference on "Islamic medicine" held in 1982 in Kuwait. Wherein a condensed view of Muslim scholars on the groupings, status and position of the sayings, deeds and directives of the Prophet (SAW) in the various books of *hadith* were presented.

To start with, there are sayings of the Prophet that are not meant to be taken as legislative authority. That is, constituting allowed or prohibited matters. Rather, they are concerned with human affairs in which the conduct of the Prophet (SAW) is more of the nature of a model than an outright canonical law. This aspect of the *hadith* covers matters relating to:

> *Human needs (eating, drinking, sleeping, etc)*
> *Experiences (medicine, agriculture, dressing, etc) Circumstances (logistics, treaties, expeditions, etc)*

Commenting further, and also quoting Sheikh Mahmoud Shaltut*, the scholar explained that the Sunnah of the Prophet is also divisible into 3 distinct categories with regards to general and specific legislation.

---

* For details see Sheikh Mahmoud Shaltur's book, *'Al-Islam Aqeeda-wa-Shari'ah (Islam as a Creed and as a Legislation)*.

Firstly, what the Prophet said in the capacity of his prophetic office as spiritual leader. These sayings include guidance on prayers, lawful and forbidden foods or acts, etc. These are considered as an extension or clarification of divine guidance and are rightly categorised as general' legislation until the Day of Judgement."

Secondly, there are prophetic statements in his capacity as a temporal leader of the Muslim community. These comprise orders given in governance, budget allocations or charities. Sayings in this case are not to be considered as legislations and no actions of this nature should be carried out without the special permission of the contemporary leader.

Thirdly, there are pronouncements of the Prophet in his judicial capacity. This are not general legislations and judgements in specific cases are not to be followed literally by everybody.

As a general rule, it is safe to say that before taking decision on a certain statement or behaviour by the Prophet, it is very important to place that action or utterance within the context of multi-dimensional capacities of the Prophet (SAW). Therefore, prophetic statement or action should be carefully judged in the light of the circumstances thereof before classifying it as Sunnah to be strictly adhered to or simply a personal way of behaviour or a judgement of a specific individual case that does not necessarily apply to all other situations.

Appreciation of this approach within the purview of this clarification will go a long way in understanding the role of the prophetic medicine, its potential and limitations, the later additions and what need to be substituted or adopted in the light of latest development in research and scholarship as prophesied by the Prophet himself. May eternal peace and blessings of Allah be upon him!

References

Abdalati, H. (1975), *Islam in Focus,* American Trust Publications, Indianapolis, USA.

Abdullahi, M. Z. (1994), Chief Host's address at the International seminar on "Islam and the Development of Science and Technology," held at Usmanu Danfodiyo University, Sokoto (UDUS), Nigeria.

Abdul Wahid, A. (1991), "Wisdom of Pork Prohibition". The Muslim Vet.

Magazine - *A Journal of Muslim Veterinary Medical Students* (MVMS) UDUS, Vol, NO.1, pp.23.

Abdul, M.O.A (1982), *The Selected Traditions of AI-Nawawi.* Islamic Publications Bureau, Lagos, Nigeria.

Abdus Salaam (1995), "Scientific Creativity in the Arab and Islamic World (Part II)." Review of Religions, London, UK.

Abubakar, A. (1992), "Prophetic Medicine." *AI-Ilm Journal of Islamic Medical Association,* Ahmadu Bello University, (ABU) Zaria, Vol. 7, NO.1 pp.24-26.

Abu Ameenah, B.P (1998), *Ibn Taimiyyah's Essay on Jinn (The Demons).* An abridged and annotated translation. International Islamic and Publishing House, Riyadh, Saudi Arabia.

Abul Fazl, M. (1993), *Steps on the Right Path: A Collection of Sayings of Prophet Muhammad.* Selected and edited by B. Aisha Lemu and Adama AI-Hasan Dolley, Islamic Education Trust, Minna, Nigeria.

Abou Azar, S.Y (n.d), *The Prophetic Medicine.* Rendered into

English from the original Arabic book *Tibbi Nabawi* of Imam Thn Qayyim AI-Jawziyya. Darnl Fikr, Beirut, Lebanon.

Adamu, U.E (1997), "Philosophy and Medical Sciences," *Al-Shifa Journal of Islamic Medical Association*, Usmanu Danfodiyo University, Sokoto (UDUS) Vol. II No.2, pp.6-8.

—— (1999). "Circumcision: A Meeting Point between Religio-Traditional and Orthodox Medicine" (unpublished work).

Adelugba, J. (n.d), *The Struggle between Islam and the West.* Agboola, A. (1998), *Textbook of Obstetrics and Gynaecology for Medical Students*, Vol. II, Pacific Printers Lagos, Nigeria.

Ahmad, T. (1994), *As-Suyuti's Medicine of The Prophet.* English translation from the original Arabic Book - *Tibbi Nabawi* of Imam Jalalud Din AbdulRahman As-Suyuti, Taha Publishers Ltd., London, UK.

Ahmad, M.B. (1982), "Islamic Faith and Treatment of Emotional Disorders." *The Muslim World League Journal.* Vol. IX NO.9 Ramadhan 1402 (July). Makka Al-Mukamamah, Saudi Arabia.

Ahmed, K. (1997), *Islam - Its Meaning and Message.* Islamic, Publication Bureau, Lagos, Nigeria.

AI-Akili, I.M. (1993), *Natural Healing with THE MEDICINE OF THE PROPHET.* Translation and Emendation of *Tibbi Nabawi* from *Zad' Al-Ma'ad* of Imam Ibn Qayyim AI-Jawziyya (1292-1350 CE). Pearl Publishing House, Philadelphia, USA.

AI-Banna, I. H. (1979), *What Is Our Message.* Islamic Publication Limited. Lahore, Pakistan.

A1-Faruq, L. L. and Y. AI-Qaradawi (1994), (com. ed) *Music: An Islamic Perspective.* Islamic Education Trust, Minna, Nigeria.

Al-Hilali, M. and M.M Khan, *Interpretation of the Meanings of the Noble Qur'{ln in the English Language.* A summarised version of AI-Tabari, Al-Qurtubi and Ibn Kathir with comments from Sahih AI-Bukhari. Damasatam Publishers and Distributors, Riyadh, Saudi Arabia.

Ali, A. Y. (1968), *Text, Translation and Commentary of the Holy Qur' an.* Light of Islam Publishers, Maiduguri, Nigeria.

Al-Kitab, N. (1997), *Patience and Gratitude.* An abridged translation of Imam Ibn Qayyim's work *Uddat as-sabirin wa dhakhiratu ash-Shakirin.* Taha Publishers, London, UK.

AI-Qaradawi, Y. (1984), *Islamic Education and HassanAl-Banna.* Holy Koran Publishing House, Beirut, Lebanon.

200 Medicine in the Qur' an and Sunnah

—— (1989), *The Lawful and the Prohibited in Islam.* AI-Tawheed Publishing Company, Lagos, Nigeria.

—— (1991), (ed). *Islamic Awakening between Rejection and Extremism.*

International Islamic Publishing House, Riyadh, Saudi Arabia.

AI-Qayrawani Ibn Abuzaid (1902), *The Risala* (Treatise on Maliki Law) - An annotated English translation from Arabic by the Catholic Priest, Joseph Kenny, Islamic Education Trust, Minna, Nigeria.

Alwani, T.J. (1995), "Islamisation of Knowledge: Yesterday and Today" *The American Journal of Islamic Social Sciences*, Vol. XII, No.1, pp.81-101.

Alwani, T.J., and Khalil I. (1991), *The Qur'an and The Sunnah: The Time-Space Factor.* IIIT, Hendon, Vrrginia, London.

Aminu, J. (1994), "The Sacred Duty To Learn and to Enquire." Paper Presented at the International Seminar on Islam and Development of Science and Technology, Us manu Danfodiyo University, Sokoto, Nigeria.

Anonymous (n.d), "Traditional Medical Practitioners and Specialists in Northern Nigeria - A Critical Analysis of Traditional Medicine and Evaluation of Possible Areas of Incorporation."

Ashraf, M. (n.d), *Sahih Muslim.* English Translation Vol. IV, Ashraf Press, Lahore, Pakistan.

Az-Zahbi, M. (1993), *Naqlil A'ada'i Baynal-Dibbi Wad-Deeni.* Daml Hadith, Jami'atu AI-Azhar - Misrah.

Badoe, E.A., E.Q., Archampong, and M.O.A. Jaja (1994) (2nd ed). *Principles and Practice of Surgery Including Pathology in the Tropics.* Assemblies of God Literature Centre Ltd. Accra, Ghana.

Balarabe, M.S.(1997), "Differences and Similarities between Islam and Christianity." A Seminar Paper Presented at the Muslim Students Society Week, Usmanu DanfodiyoUniversity, Sokoto (UDUS), Nigeria.

Bashir, A. (1998), "Contributions of Muslims to the Field of Medical Sciences", *Islamapharm - Journal of the Muslim Pharmaceutical Students Association*, ABU, Zaria, Vol. 1, No.1, pp. 8-10.

Begum Aisha Bawamy, *Islam: The Religion of all Prophets -* An Abridged and Combined Edition of "Charms ofIslam" and "Islam our Choice." Waqf Publishers, Karachi, Pakistan.

Bucaille, M. (1979), *The Bible, The Qur'an and Modern Science.* North American Trust Publication, Indianapolis, USA.

Bugaje, U. (1995), "Some Contributions of the Sokoto Caliphate Scholars To the Study of Medicine." Paper Presented at the Annual Conference of the Islamic Medical Association, UDUS, Nigeria.

Carpaner, M., Kamali A. *etal(1999)*, "Rates of IDV Transmission within Marriage in Rural Uganda in Relation to the mv Sera-Status of the Partners," AIDS 13:1083-1089.

Chamberlain, nv.p. (1995), (ed). *Obstetrics by Ten Teachers* (16th Edition). Edward Arnorld, London, UK.

Dauda, Y. (1999), *Islam, Science and Survival of Mankind.* Iman Services Ltd. (Publishers), Lagos, Nigeria

Deen Digest. *A Monthly Journal of Islamic Thoughts and Views.* Vol. V, No.9, Jan/Feb 2000 (Shawwal/Dhul Qidah 1420).

Derek Llewellyn Jones, *Every Woman - A Gynaecological Guide for Life* .. Safari Books (Export) Limited, London, Channel Island, UK.

Doi, A. I. (1970), *Introduction to the Hadith.* Islamic Publications Bureau, Lagos, Nigeria.

—— (1981), *Introduction to the Qur'an.* Arewa Books Ltd., Ibadan, Nigeria.

—— (1982), *Prayersfrom the Qur'an and Sunnah.* Gaskiya Corporation Ltd., Zaria, Nigeria.

Elkadi, A. (1991), "Health and Healing in the Qur'an." *Th~ Muslim Woman Journal of Federated Organisation of Muslim Women Associations of Nigeria*, Vol, No.3.

Faisal, A (1997), *Natural Instincts* (Islamic Psychology). Darnl Islam Publishers, London, UK.

Farid, A H. (n.d), *Prayers of Muhammad*. Islamic Publications Bureau, Lagos, Nigeria.

Faris, A.W. (1966), *The Book of Knowledge*. (2nd ed). English translation and notes adopted from *Ihya 'u Ulumuddin* of Imam AI-Ghazzali, Ashraf Press, Lahore, Pakistan.

Field, C.M.A (n.d), *The Confessions of AI-Ghazzali*. Ashraf Press Ltd., Lahore, Pakistan.

Fodio, Abdullahi bn, *Masalihal Insani AI-Mutadalliqa bil Adyani Wal Abdani*.

Galadanci, B.S.(n.d), "Islamisation of the Natural Sciences - Myth or Reality." Paper Presented at the Muslim Forum Seminar on Islamisation of Knowledge at Bayero University, Kano, Nigeria.

— (2000), "Islamisation of Knowledge: Concept and Core Issues." *Al-Irshad - A Quarterly Magazine of the National Islamic Centre*. Vol. ill, No.1, Jan., 2000. (Ram. 1420) pp. 1-5 and 7.

Gayi, H.A (1998), "Consanguineous Marriage: Its Medico-Social Problems." *The Likita-Journal of the Kebbi State. Medical Students Association*, UDUS. Vol. I, NO.1 NovlDec.

Goerlnger, G. c., A A Zindani and M. A Ahmed (1992), "Description of Human Development: *Izam* and *Lahm* Stages," *In* Zindani et al (ed). *Human Development as Described in the Qur'an and Sunnah*. World Muslim League Press, Makkah, Saudi Arabia.

— (1992), "Some Aspects of the Historical Progress in Embryology through the Ages," *Ibid.*

Guschier A., G. R., Giles and AR. Moosa (n.d) (ed). *Essential Surgical Practice* (3rd Edition). Butte worth Heinemann Ltd., Oxford.

Guyton, A C., and E.H, Hall (n.d). *Textbook of Medical Physiology,* W.B. Saunders Company, Philadelphia, Pennsylvania, USA

Holland, M. (1983), *Inner Dimensions of Islamic Worship.* Translated from the *Ihya* of Imam AI-Ghazzali. The Islamic Foundation, London, UK.

— (n.d). *Duties of Brotherhood in Islam.* Translated from the *Ihya* of Imam Al-Ghazzali. Islamic Foundation, London, UK.

Holy Bible (Old & New Testaments), King James Version (1972), Thomas Nelson Inc, New York, USA.

Holy Bible (The New Testament), The Gideons International (1979), Thomas Nelson Inc., New York, USA.

Holy Qur'an: English Translation of the Meanings and Commentary: Revised and Edited by the Presidency of Islamic Research, 1FT A, Call and Guidance, King Fahd Holy Qur' an Printing Complex, Madina, Saudi Arabia.

Hussain, S.S. (1992), *A Young Muslim's Guide To Religions in the World.* Bangladesh Institute of Islamic Thought, Dacca.

Ibrahim M.T.a. (1997), "Family Planning between Rejection and Acceptance in Islam." Risalatus-Shifa - *A Journal of National Association of Muslim and Paramedical Students* Vol. 1, No. 1, pp. 28-31.

Idris, M. (n.d) (ed), *Muwatta Imam Malik*. English translation, Diwan Press, Norwich, England.

Imam Al-Ghazzali, A.H. *Revivification of Religious Sciences*. English translation by Maulana Fazhul-Karim Vol. I and II. Taj Company, New Delhi, India.

Iqbal, M. (n.d), *The Reconstruction of Religious Thought in Islam*. Ashraf Press, Lahore, Pakistan.

Irving, T.B. (Ta'alim Ali) (1979), *Islam Resurgent: The Islamic World Today*. Islamic Publications Bureau, Lagos, Nigeria.

Isah, H. (1998). "Honey - A Natural Cure from Allah." *Islamapharm Magazine of the Pharmaceutical Muslim Students Society of Nigeria*, ABU, Zaria, Nigeria, Vol. I. No.1, pp.19.

Islamic Medical Association of Uganda (1998), *AIDS Education through Imams: A Spiritually Motivated Community Effort in Uganda*.

Islamic Education Trust (1992), *Misconception About Islam*. I.E.T., Minna, Nigeria.

Iwegbu, C.G (1988), *Principles and Management of Acute Orthopedic Trauma*. Institute of Education Press, ABU, Zaria, Nigeria.

Izetbegovic, AA (1989), *Islam between East and West*. American Trust Publications, Indianapolis, USA

Jude, U. O. (1994), "The Relevance of the Concept of Spiritual Health." *The Medicare Medical Journal*, Vol. 5, No.10, pp. 11.

Jumba, AM.Y. (1994), "The Contributions of Islam to Science and Technology." Paper Presented at the International seminar on Islam and the Development of Science and Technology held at Usmanu Danfodiyo University, Sokoto, Nigeria.

Junaidu, A U. (2000), "Zoonoses and Attainment of Health for All Beyond 2000." Paper Presented at the Opening Ceremony of the Annual Veterinary Week, UDUS, Nigeria.

Kagimu M. Marum, E. and Serwadda, D (1995), ''Planning and Evaluating Strategies for AIDS Health Education Interventions in the Muslims Community in Uganda." *AIDS Education Prevention* 10 (3), 215-228, pp. 7,1021.

Kagimu M., Maru, E. and Wabiwire-Mangen E, Nakyanjo, N., Walakira, Y. and Hogyle J. (1998), "Evaluation of the Effectiveness of AIDS Health Education Interventions in the Muslim Community in Uganda." *AIDS Education Prevention* 10 (3), 215-228.

Kani, AM. (1994), "Muslims Attitude towards Science and Technology in the Post-Industrial Era", *Risalatus Shifa* Vol. 1, Edition No.1, pp.14-19.

Kasarawa, AB. (1995), "Challenges of Modern Science to the Muslims."

Paper Presented at the National Conference of the National Association of Muslim Medical and Paramedical Students Held at ABU, Zaria.

Kaura, J. M. (1994), "Integration of Muslim Women in the Development of Science and Technology." Paper Presented at the International Seminar on Islam and the Development of Science and Technology Held at Usmanu Danfodiyo University, Sokoto, Nigeria.

Khalid, S. (1994), "Science and Epistemological crisis: The Need for an Islamic alternative." Paper Presented at the

International Seminar on "Islam and the Development of Science and Technology" Held at Usmanu Danfodiyo University, Sokoto, Nigeria.

Khalil, I. (1991), *Islamisation of Knowledge: A Methodology.* IIIT, Herdon, Vrrginia, London.

Khan, M. M. (1985), *Sahih Bukhari.* Arabic-English Translation. Vol. VII and IX. Daml Arabia Publishing, Printing and Distribution, Beirut, Lebanon.

Khan, M. A. (1987), *The Right Path.* Translation of *Al-Murajat* of Abdal Husayn Sharaf AI-Din AI-Musawi. Zahra Publications, USA.

Lemu, A.S. (n.d), *A Book of Fasting.* Islamic Education Trust, Minna, Nigeria.

Magaji, A.A. (1997), "Diseases of Animals Communicable to Man and The Need for National Public Awareness and Control." Paper Presented at the 8th Annual Veterinary Week of the Association of Veterinary Medical Students, UDUS, Vol. 1, Edition, NO.1, pp. 44.

Mahmud, A. (1978), *The Creed of Islam.* World of Islam Festival Trust, London (1978).

Malamba, S.S, Wagner, H. *et al* (1994), "Risk Factors for HIV- I Infection Among Adults in a Rural Uganda Community: A Case Control Study." *AIDS 8:253-57.*

Manga, U.H. (1998), "Killer Disease from Dogs" *The Likita-Journal* of Kebbi State Medical Students Association, UDUS Vol. 1, Edition, NO.1, pp.16.

Mann, C.Y., and RC.G. Russel (1992), (ed). *Bailey & Love's Short Practice of Surgery.* (Revised) 21st Edition. Chapman and Hall, London, UK.

Marshall, E.J, A.A. Zindani and M.A. Ahmed (1992),

"Description of Human Development: The *Nutfah* Stage," In A. A. Zindani *et al* (ed), *Human Development as Described in the Qur'an and Sunnah*. World Muslim League Press, Makkah, Saudi Arabia.

Mikailu, A.S. (1995), "Islamisation of Social Sciences in Nigeria – Problems and Prospects." *The American Journal of Islamic Social Sciences* Vol. XII, No.1, Spring.

—— (1996), "Islamisation of Knowledge in Nigeria: Problems and Prospects" A Paper Presented during the Workshop on Islamisation of Knowledge at the Institute of Administration, ABU, Zaria.

Miller G (nd), *The Amazing Qur'an*. Islamic Education Trust, Minna, Nigeria.

Mohammed, Y. (1994), "Islamisation of Knowledge: A Critique." *The American Journal of Islamic Social Sciences* Vol. II, No.2 Summer. Published by Association of Muslim Social Scientists and International Institute of Islamic Thought.

Moore, Keith L. (1982), *Developing Human: Clinically Oriented Anatomy* (3rd edition). W.B. Sauders Company, Philadelphia, USA.

—— (1986), "A Scientist's Interpretation of References to Embryology in the Qur'an." *Journal of Islamic Medical Association.*

Moore Keith, L. andAA Zindani (1983), *The Developing Human with Islamic Additions*. Dar-al Qibah for Islamic Literature, Jeddah, Saudi Arabia.

Moore, K.L., AA Zindani and M. A Ahmed (1992a), "New Terms for Classifying Human Development," In Zindani *et al* (ed) *Human Development as Described in the Qur'an and Sunnah*. World Muslim League Press,

Makkah, Saudi Arabia.

—— (1992b), "Description of Human Development: *Alaqah* and *Mudghah* Stages," *Ibid.*

Mora, M. S. (1992), "The Contribution of Muslim Scholars to Medicine," *Al-Ilm* Journal ofisiamic Medical Association, ABU, Zaria Vol. 7, No.1, pp. 27-30.

Muhammad, A.Y.(1994), "Islamic Perspectives on Medical and Paramedical Codes of Ethics." Paper Presented at the International Seminar on Islam and the Development of Science and Technology held at Usmanu Danfodiyo University, Sokoto, Nigeria.

Muhammad, A. Y. (1995), "Islamic Perspectives on Medical and Paramedical Ethics." Paper Presented at the Annual Health Week of the Islamic Medical Association, UDUS.

Muhammad, H. (1995), "The Holy Prophet As a Medical Man." *Al-Shifa Journal of Islamic Medical Association,* UDUS Vol. II, No.2.

Mungadi, A. I. (1997), "Smoking and Health." Adopted from the original Seminar Paper "Surgery and Smoking" Presented during the Annual Scientific Conference of the Association of Resident Doctors, University ofllorin, Dorin, Nigeria.

Murad, M. (1989), *Islam in Brief.* Islamic Call Centre, Lagos, Nigeria. Murray R. K., D. K. Granner and P. A. Mayer and V. W. Rodwell *(1999), Harper's Biochemistry* (24th edition). Printice Hall, International Inc., New Jersey, USA.

Nadwi, *S.A. Muhammad Rasulullahi (The Life of the Prophet Muhammad).* Translated by Mohiuddin Ahmed and Academy of Islamic Research and Publications,

Luckvow, India.

Nancy Roper's (1995), *Pocket Medical Dictionary* (14th Edition). Churchill Living Stone London, UK.

National AIDS and STD Control Programme. *Handbook on HIV Infection and AIDS for Health Workers,* Lagos, 1992.

Neal, M. J. *Medical Pharmacology* at a *Glance.* Oxford Blackwell Scientific Publications, London, UK.

Nigerian Journal of Medicine. Vol. VII, NO.2, April-June 1998, Published by the National Association of Resident Doctors of Nigeria.

Nigerian Journal of Pharmacy. Vol. 31, Jan-Feb., 2000. Published by Pharmaceutical Society of Nigeria.

Njoku, C.H. (1999), "Smoking and Your Health", *Likita - Journal of Usmanu Danfodiyo University Medical Students Association* (UDUMSA), Vol. III, No.1, pp.

Njozi, H. M. (1989), *The Sources of the Qur'an - A Critical Review of Authorship Theories.* AI-Balagh Publishers, Lagos, Nigeria.

Num, A J., Kengeya-Kayondo, J. F. *et al* (1994), "Risk Factor for HIV-I Infectjon in Adults in a Rural Uganda Community: A Population-Study.'~ *AIDS 8:81-86.*

Nurudeen, O.A (1998), "Pig not for Human Use - Islam and Veterinary Science's View." *The Voice of Islam - Journal of the Muslim Students Society,* UDUS, Vol.1, No.1, pp.32.

Okonofua, F. E. (1997), "Management of Infertility in Mrica." *Dokita Medical* Journal - Proceeds of the 1997 Annual Symposium of *Dokita* Editorial Board, University College Hospital, Ibadan, pp.10-20.

Parry, E.H.O. (1984), *Principles and Practice of Medicine in*

Africa. (2nd Edition). Oxford University Press, London, UK.

Persaud, T.Y.N., AA. Zindani and M. A Ahmed (1992a), "Description of Human Development: *Nash 'ah* Stage", In AA Zindani *et al* (ed), *Human Development as Described in the Qur'an and Sunnah,* World Muslim League Press, Makkah, Saudi Arabia.

- (1992b), "Human Development After the Forty-second Day." *Ibid.* Pickthall, M. Marmaduke, *The Meaning of the Glorious Koran.* An explanatory English translation of the holy Qur'an. Islamic Publication Bureau, Lagos, Nigeria

Pratt, R. J. (1995), *HIV and AIDS: A Strategy for Nursing Care.* (4th Edition), Edward Arnold Publishers.

Qutb, Sayyid (1978), *Milestones.* International Islamic Federation of Muslim Student Organisations, Salimiah, Kuwait.

—— (1979), *Islam - The Misunderstood Religion.* Islamic Publication Limited., Lahore, Pakistan.

Rahim, A. (1992), *Islamic History.* Islamic Publication Bureau. Lagos, Nigeria.

Rahimudin, M. (1985), *Muwatta Imam Malik.* English translation, Photocopying and Electronic Centre, Beirut, Lebanon.

Rana Din, M., *What is Islam.* Taha Publishers London.

Rashid, I.H. (1987), *Quranology - The Practical Solution* to *the World s Problems and Crisis.*

Rauf, M. A. (1982), *The Sacred Texts of Islam: AI-Qur'an and Al-Hadith.* Islamic Publication Bureau, Lagos, Nigeria.

Research: *The Bayer Scientific Magazine.* 7th Edition. Lever Kusen, Germany.

Roberts, M.B.V. *Biology: A Functional Approach.* (4th Edition), Thomas Nelson and Sons Ltd., Surrey, U.K.

Roderick, A. C., W. M. Alexandar, B. M. Peter and S. Z. Ghazi (1989), *Pathology: The Mechanisms of Disease* (2nd Edition). The c.v. Mosby Company, Missouri, USA.

Ruth Koenigsberg's Illustrated Churchill's *Medical Dictionary (1989),* Churchill's Livingstone Inc, New York, USA.

Sabir, A.A. (1995), "Honey - A Natural Cure from *Allah".* *Al-Shifa'a.*

A Journal of the Islamic Medical Association, UDUS. Vol. II, No.2, pp. 20. .

Sadler, T.W, (1985), *Longmans Medical Embryology* (8th Edition) Williams and Wilkins, Baltimore.

Sambo, A. S., A. S. Mikailu, 1. M. Kaura, M. Tabiu and N. M. Abubakar (1998), (ed). *Islam and Development of Science and Technology.* (Seminar Series No.1), Islamic Research Centre, Sokoto, Nigeria.

Sayyid, Abul Ala Maududi (1960), *Towards Understanding Islam.*

International Islamic Publishing House, Riyadh, Saudi Arabia.

SayyidLari, M. M. (1988), "God, Human Knowledge and Science," AI-*Tawheed - A Quarterly Journal of Islamic Thought and Culture.* Vol. V, Nos. 3 and 4, Rajab - Dhul al-Hijjah 1408, pp 85-152.

Shariff, M. M. (1963), *History of Muslim Philosophy.* Vol. I, Otto harrussowitz Wiesbaden, Lahore, Pakistan.

Shehu, S. (1996), "The Islamic Vision of Knowledge - Its Implication and Significance to the Islamisation of Knowledge Programme." Paper Presented at a Seminar on Islamisation of Knowledge, Bayero University, Kano, Nigeria.

—— (2000), "Islamising the Educational System: Towards an Alternative Education, Theory and Agenda for the Muslim Ummah in Nigeria." Paper Presented at a Two Day National Workshop on Islamisation of knowledge at the Usmanu Danfodiyo University, Sokoto, Nigeria.

Siddiqi, A. H. (1971), Sahih Muslim: English Translation Vol. III, Darnl Arabia, Publishing, Printing and Distribution, Beirut, Lebanon.

The Journal of Islamic Medical Association of North America. Vol. 32, No.2, April 2000, pp 49-84.

The Reminder Vol. n, Issue No.1, June 2000. *A Newsletter of the Islamic Medical Association of Uganda*, Kampala, Uganda.

Wan Daud, W.M.N. (1989), *The Concept of Knowledge in Islam*. University Press, Cambridge, UK.

Waqf 1khlas, *Islam and Christianity*. Publication No. 12, Islamic Seminary, Istanbul, Thrkey.

Yusuf, H. M. (1998), *Anatomy of the Qur'an: Fact or Fallacy?* Thrash Islamic Publications Centre Limited, Lagos, Nigeria.

Zayyid, M.Y: (1980), *An English Translation of the Meaning of the Qur'an*. Dar-AI-Choura Publishers, Beirut, Lebanon.

Zindani, A. A., M. A. Ahmed, M. B. Tobin and T.V.N. Persaud (1992), *Human Development as Described in the Qur' an and Sunnah*. Muslim World League Press, MakkahAI-Mukarramah, Saudi Arabia.

Zindani, A. A., M. A. Ahmed and J. L. Simpson (1992), "Embryogenesis and Human Development in the First Forty Days" *Ibid.*

INDEX

297

101, 110, 112, 120, 127-
128, 130-132, 136-143,
146-147, 150, 159, 161,
165, 167,170-174, 177,
180-184, 193, 195, 199,
201-202, 205-206, 210,
212, 215, 217, 220, 222-
227, 229, 232, 236-237,
270-271, 281-282
- Jesus (AS), 174–175
- Job (AS), 73, 160
- Muhammad (SAW), 1,
  6-7, 9-10–11, 15, 16,
  19-21, 25-27, 29-31
- Sulaiman (AS), 158, 172
- Zachariah (AS), 90. 195
Prophets of God, 15
Prophet's
- companions, 31, 167,
  225
- injunctions, 42
- prayer, 195
Prophetic
- guidance on medicine,
  236
- medicine, 67, 81, 236,
  277-282
Prophylaxis, 216
Psychoanalysis, 96
Psychological
- counseling, 98
- disorders, 53, 271
- terror, 186
Psychotherapy, 96-105

Qada wa qadr (destiny and
  predestination), 144
Qadr (concept of
  predestination), 262
Qadr (predestination), 203
Qarar (place of settlement),
  138
Qatada bn Al-Numan, 173

Qur'anic
- recitation , 106
- and supplication,
  61
- and Sunnah, 6
- injunctions, 9-10, 23
- message, 10, 271
- passages, 270
- verses, 204
- wisdom, 193

Rabies, 118
Recreational activities, 48-49
Religion education, 200
Religious
- knowledge, 16, 156,
  258
- obligation, 231
- psychotherapy, 107
- traditional medicine,
  37
Remedy with milk, 84–85
Restraining force, 98
Right
- medicine, 26, 151 216
- and obligations,
  270
Rights
- of children, 201
- of inheritance, 194
Risala (message), 10
Rizq(provision), 203
Robinson, Victor, 240
Royal jelly, 71-72
Rufaida, 223
Ruqya, 106
- prayer, 85
- treatment of diseases,
  91, 93
Sa'id bn Abi Waqqas (RA) 79
Sabr (patience for bearance,
  fortitude), 105
Sacred (Shar'iyah), 23